ENERGY HEALING

ENERGY HEALING
A Surprising Form of Medicine

Wilhelm Johannes Frinta

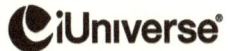

ENERGY HEALING
A SURPRISING FORM OF MEDICINE

iUniverse books may be ordered through booksellers or by contacting:

iUniverse
1663 Liberty Drive
Bloomington, IN 47403
www.iuniverse.com
1-800-Authors (1-800-288-4677)

Because of the dynamic nature of the Internet, any web addresses or links contained in this book may have changed since publication and may no longer be valid. The views expressed in this work are solely those of the author and do not necessarily reflect the views of the publisher, and the publisher hereby disclaims any responsibility for them.

Any people depicted in stock imagery provided by Getty Images are models, and such images are being used for illustrative purposes only. Certain stock imagery © Getty Images.

ISBN: 978-1-5320-4979-8 (sc)
ISBN: 978-1-5320-4980-4 (e)

Print information available on the last page.

iUniverse rev. date: 06/18/2018

DEDICATION

This book is dedicated to the thousands of patients who have overcome all their prejudices and been able to allow their ailments to be treated with *energy healing*. Their faith in this new and surprising technique has allowed them to experience life-enhancing improvements at physical, psychic and spiritual levels.

"The most beautiful thing we can experience is the mysterious. It is the source of all true art and science. He to whom the emotion is a stranger, who can no long pause to wonder and stand wrapped in awe, is as good as dead —his eyes are closed. The insight into the mystery of life, coupled though it be with fear, has also given rise to religion. To know what is impenetrable to us really exists, manifesting itself as the highest wisdom and the most radiant beauty, which our dull faculties can comprehend only in their most primitive forms—this knowledge, this feeling is at the center of true religiousness."

Albert Einstein

CONTENTS

TO THE READER

This book is the fruit of the ethical commitment I made as a therapistsome years ago, which consists in sharing with each of you my experience and my knowledge of the world of *healing*, particularly as regards its immense potential to servemedical science. By inviting you to read this book my aim is precisely to broaden our knowledge of the phenomenon of *healing*. It follows that this work has no commercial motivation; rather, its purpose is to assist the reader towards the fullest possible understanding of the many options provided by the therapies of healing, as practiced throughout the world by many highly respected and highly talented professionals as they pit their own methods in the perennial struggle of man versus disease.

Wilhelm Johannes Frinta

PRESENTATION

Energy Healing, a surprising form of Medicine, by Dr. Frinta, introduces us to a new medicine for our millennium, because what he proposes in this book reaches beyond the limits of conventional anatomy and physiology to the fields of trans-dimensional physiology and physiopathology, insofar aswe find ourselves, when he speaks of "therapeutic vibrational frequencies that interact with the patients' vibrational fields in either brain or tissue", faced with aspects in a different dimension to those of the familiar field of organic matter.

The therapeutic proposals sketched by Dr. Frinta in this book invite us to look at the matter-energy interface as an active, dynamic and interactive dimensionality of all the physiological levels of the human body where vibration information is processed and where the workings of health and disease are revealed.

It is also a work born of clinical practice, because it is not a theoretical compilation, but springs from the therapeutic experience of many years of working and experimenting in the fields of subtle energy, fields that are as yet little understood by modern science, which lacks the technology for accurate quantitative evaluation of them. What is important here are the clear results of the interaction of these fields of this energy with the patients who benefit from it. Dr. Frinta states that "healing is not only of the body but is multidimensional", so the concept of healing acquiresa deeper meaning, and this is fundamental insofar as each patient, doctor, health worker and society in general must eventually come to a full understanding of the fact that "true healing comes from within the person and moves outwards according to processes that involve profound dynamics of the psyche according to the continuous effort to perfect the self and to achieve the full harmony of the soul". Thus it is that, depending on our level of evolution and understanding of the laws of the universe, we will either continue for a long time to seek healing through processes outside of ourselves, or we will begin to follow the path of searching for interior peace, so essential to our physiological balance and thus to our true health and wholeness.

From a philosophical point of view this work barely sketches out the role played by reincarnation, the law of cause and effect as regards the origin and development of the many diseases that afflict humanity, as also as regards the level of improvement or recuperation achievable by patients through vibrational healings. These concepts have enriched Dr. Frinta's cultural stock as he has faced the challenges needed to make his therapy available in our society, challenges overcome by the virtues expressed in his personality such as his spirit of service, his desire to work without self interest for the good of his patients, his discipline and total dedication to his therapy, as witnessed in the pioneering work he carried out some ten years ago in the San Rafael Hospital in Facatativá, Colombia, where over a number of years his care for several thousand patients was provided without remuneration.

Dr. Frinta tells us also that "the loss of the notion of time and space" is the main indication he has noticed in his patients, as something strange that they have experienced during the therapies; this fact being of the greatest significance if we take into account the parameters mentioned by Dr. Larry Dossey in his book entitled *Re-inventing Medicine*, in which he talks of eras in medicine. Era I is Mechanical medicine, Era II is medicine of the mind-body synergy, and in Era III he places the medicine of not localizing the mind, since it has no place in time or space, and within this last era of medicine he situates all those therapies where the effects produced by conscience can involve two or more people. He tells us that the implications for medicine of this fact are very profound, and that the faculty of non-location of the mind offers us a means to help us cure each other, thereby making health and disease a collective problem. We believe that those patients who have lost the notion of time and space are those best able to improve or be cured, since by being in a state of non localized conscience they are able to achieve the most significant therapeutic effects. Thus we can affirm that Dr. Frinta is undoubtedly in Era III of medicine, the surprising medicine of the future which is with us in the present thanks to his valuable work, contributing towards today's science the many demonstrations of the effectiveness of his *vibrational healing.*

Fabio Villarraga B.
MD, National University of Colombia

PROLOGUE

My decision to write this book is not merely the inevitable consequence of my desire to share with you the experience of treating thousands of patients who had faith in the value of my therapy and of the astounding potential that *healing*, based on the use of vibrational frequencies, offers the world of medicine.

The work you have in your hands is above all the result of long and deep reflection, due above all to my enthusiastic desire that the reader should know the nature of *healing* in all its dimensions, both as a successful therapy in the struggle against disease and in the choice of life that this implies in relation to our physical, mental and spiritual wellbeing. It is of course a further contribution to my efforts to overcome the great dearth of knowledge that mistakenly places *healing* in a mysterious and intangible context, thereby making it unintelligible to the layman.

Talabisms contribute nothing to the concretization of the right we all have to know the benefits of *healing* as an area of medicine that is able, at times, despite the unjust suspicion with which it is still viewed, to replace costly invasive treatments that include indiscriminate prescription of chemical drugs, with their harmful side effects, and every kind of surgical intervention. Conscious of the challenge implied in presenting the reader with material involving a high level of science, this work is written in clear and simple language that invites the reader to broaden his awareness of the human organism's ability to fight disease if we allow the energies of the cosmos to work with us. The pages you are about to read are likewise a means of approaching the world of *healing* in every sense, with its potential and its limitations, and to do so without any form of fanaticism. I mean to give the reader all the information I have at my disposal to encourage understanding of this therapy based on frequencies, whose origin, though still a mystery to science, belongs nevertheless to a reality which will undoubtedly be revealed to us in the near future.

Likewise, these pages do not aim to raise false expectations about the curative powers of *healing*, a therapy often mistakenly identified with miracles and all kinds of supernatural experiences belonging to a realm that defies our understanding and, as will be evident throughout the book, in no way resembles vibrational *healing* based on non magnetic frequencies that I have to define as being of cosmic origin.

Finally, I hope this work may help clarify the confused panorama that has grown out of the increasing and legitimate criticisms of the rigid orthodoxy of conventional medicine administered by the health systems—themselves equally rigid and orthodox—which seem to reflect the economic interests of the large multinational corporations of the pharmaceutical industry.

It is appropriate to make this clarification owing to the suspicion engendered by these criticisms and which over the past years have given rise to the editorial *boom* of the ill named "alternative medicine", several of whose works do indeed appear to be bent on justifying its efficiency and validity on the basis of the prejudiced disqualification of all other therapies.

More than patients, we need readers able to develop a more open mentality that enables us to meet the challenges of the future, and this obliges us to put aside that slight of words whereby the patient is still seen as a passive agent and not as a subject who needs to participate actively in the design of his health systems.

INTRODUCTION

In 1950, the year I was born, Salzburg, in western Austria, with 105.000 inhabitants on either side of the Salzach river, was a city obsessed with the reconstruction of its ancient cathedral, whose presbytery and one of its towers had been destroyed by the bombing that shook the city in the last days of the Second World War.

The stony outlines of its castles, of its many gothic and baroque churches, of its medieval fortresses and imperial and archbishop's palaces are an unlikely indication that, rather than in the alpine peace of Salzburg on the other side of the world, my *raison d'être*, the practice of my profession and my love for knowledge of energies as the reliable base for treating a variety of diseases, would be rooted in Colombia of the early 1980s, a troubled chapter in the life of that Latin American country.

Until then, my life had been typical of an adolescent in Europe. When I completed secondary studies I had no idea what lay in wait for me. I did not know what to study or where to study it, so one can imagine that I was not even sure I wanted to continue studying. I was in fact in a state of some anguish, yet I overcame this state almost unwittingly when, after attempts at Sociology, Psychology and even Law, I decided to read Medicine at Innsbruck University.

Towards the end of 1972, when I was nearly 22, I felt I was old enough to begin new studies so, before taking a step that I might have regretted, and sensing that I probably had little choice but to aim for a respected career that would guarantee a conventional life for a young Austrian with a Catholic education, I found in Innsbruck, in western Austria, the conditions that would lead to this new life.

I was ready, at the time, to become a conventional doctor in my country, in a society where a consulting room, a tensiometer and a stethoscope would symbolize a prosperous and traditional standing in any of our cities in the foothills of the Alps. Innsbruck University, surrounded by mountains that seemed to protect us from misfortune, was enough to give me the encouragement and the confidence I needed to feel sure that I would achieve these aims. After two semesters I felt really sure of myself:—though I needed to work at the week-ends to pay for my studies, nothing seemed complicated in that city, and my aim to become a conventional doctor was being confirmed. I was very sure of the orthodox calling that would await me at the end of my studies, and what I could expect once I was in possession of my doctor's diploma, with the prestige to fulfill the dream of belonging to a highly respected professional body.

However, it was precisely my delight in this prestige that warned me about the temptation to become not just an excellent doctor but perhaps someone who looked on others with arrogance, particularly as regards patients who are often looked down on by traditional doctors, convinced that only they understand disease. This arrogance is not diminishing: it is unfortunately all too common among medical practitioners today.

But my fear that I might become a petulant medical practitioner was not the only factor; I was moved also by my interest in anthropology, in history and in philosophy, so that I became more convinced that I had a mission, and that this might be fulfilled in other latitudes. So I looked towards Latin America, first in Mexico and then in Colombia, where I arrived in March of 1983, and where my life became very different to what it had been until that moment.

I found myself in a context of enormous poverty, exclusion, social inequality and every type of problem coexisting with elites that resisted any change in the social order, and this affected me deeply and gave me a profound motivation to try by any means at my disposal to make the situation in the country better.

My first years in Colombia were immensely happy. I was at peace as I practiced my profession along orthodox lines, but felt fulfilled because my patients were Latin Americans. The warmth, friendliness and hospitality of Colombians is something that always impresses foreigners. I soon felt at home with their gentleness, politeness and simplicity, especially that of the most humble and needy among them, and found my fulfillment in giving them my fullest dedication over a period of several years.

However, my thinking was shaped along new lines by a series of events that occurred towards the end of the 1980s. This did not happen by chance or suddenly. It was the result of growing contact with people who, in keeping with a Latin American tradition, held a less materialistic worldview than that which dominated in Europe and was so resistant to accepting the existence of things intangible to our senses.

Little by little I became involved with people whose views on life and how to face its realities were different from my own, including a vision of medicine that challenged my rigid belief in what I had learned up to that point. With what solid arguments could I now defend the inflexibility of our conventional medical focus? Was not this the focus that could rightly be called traditional? And if by traditional we understand that which opposes innovation, then should we not ask if innovation is not the natural source of evolution in human knowledge?

With more questions than answers, without hysteria or fanaticism, I continued to consider these new perceptions which challenged my dependence—itself undoubtedly irrational—on a faculty medicine that despised, and still despises today, all contributions that do not stem from the material world of tangible things in the literal sense of these words.

From then on I experienced confusion, as my humanist education and the Catholic foundation of my religious formation struggled with a mental openness that would allow me to accept knowledge other than that of the dogmas and traditions they represented as uniquely valid.

One example of this was the subject of reincarnation. It was frankly difficult to suddenly accept an alternative to the dogma of resurrection proclaimed by the Council of Nicaea, whereby I would admit, on the one hand, the possibility that "body and soul do not exist simultaneously but rotate their existence on a scale of perennial movement towards perfection", or that both notions are combined so that what is physical or sensory is part of a sort of testing period for the spiritual dimension, which itself governs all other dimensions of human existence.

It was a matter of years, not months, before my mind could shape the possibility of accepting this principle of reincarnation as the guiding axis of life, and this undoubtedly implied that I was open to further questions, many of them still unanswered. Though we are unsure how, when and why reincarnation occurs, we are nevertheless aware that it allows us to reinterpret life in a way that benefits our physical, mental and spiritual existence.

In effect, matter, reason and spirit, probably the most accepted manifestations of human existence in the course of history, constitute a triad which can—why not?—benefit each of us throughout our material or cellular life, and in my opinion this could clash with the idea of more complex dimensions in which matter, because it is the transitory or mortal part of our being, is hierarchically inferior to spirit, because this is the immortal part.

We may have no doubts about this, as occurs with me. However, it would be to take things a lot further were we to pretend that, by accepting this superiority, the spiritual level of the human being might play a part, whatever that may be, in man's perennial struggle to overcome disease on the path to achieving happiness.

Though this is in no way a treatise of philosophy, I believe that reflection on themes such as this should be part of the formation of doctors in every part of the world and every cultural context because their work, as we know, is aimed at preventing and combating disease and promoting a better quality of life for us humans.

Such contact with other ways of thinking will surely broaden our reasoning awareness in the face of life and death, insofar as this perception could allow us to see these no longer as something absolute but rather in more relative terms. Thus if we stop thinking of life as something absolute, based on our always juxtaposing it with the irrefutable fact of death, and likewise if we remove death from that same absolute condition, then we become able to achieve a balance where the material and spiritual dimensions of our beings interact in benefit of our existence.

Of course, since, from the perspective of reason, life precedes death, then the anguish of the awareness of death can and should be dealt with by changing our conception of this apparently immutable order, substituting for it a cycle in which spirit precedes life and life is followed in turn by spirit.

This balance that I believe exists between life and death has implications for the practical existence of human beings. Nevertheless, the limits of my personal existence prevent me from being sure of all I have humbly reflected on from the basis of my medical, physical and humanist perspectives. So the reader needs to understand clearly that what I have contributed here is the result of personal reflections based on my knowledge and experience, on which I have based my personal conclusions which may certainly be different from those reached in all freedom by others after they have read these lines.

However, alongside these intimate conclusions I must still place my trust in the triumph of these new perspectives of medicine that are holistic, integral and indeed supra-dimensional, if we are to borrow the precise word used by Dr. Fabio Villaraga. Acupuncture is a clear example of how new notions have been accepted in Western medicine and have come to configure, on the basis of this acceptance, though not without difficulties, a path of healthy coexistence between allopathic medicine, on the one hand, i.e. medicine that views treatment through the prescription of synthetic drugs that attack the symptoms of disease, and medicine incorrectly named "alternative", on the other, of which acupuncture is nowadays one of the most accepted techniques for combating disease. Thus it is that acupuncture, a legendary therapy of Chinese medicine, is now beginning to be financed alongside others by public health systems, on a similar legal basis whereby it is no longer a model that is "alternative" or residual to conventional medical practice, but is a technique fully recognized whereby a human organism forms an integral part of a balance between the micro-cosmos and the macro-cosmos.

The search for this aim supposes its merging with another balance: that which springs from the relationship between the mental and the organic spheres, whereby the patient progresses towards sanity by means of regular physical exercise combined with a healthy diet and a positive mental attitude. This psycho-physical balance involves a nucleus of disease prevention and healing that for centuries was ignored in the West in favour of allopathic conceptions—from the Greek *allo*=other, and *pathos*=disease—an etymology that condenses the philosophy of this classical medicine which holds that drugs of synthesis are the only way to combat symptoms and manifestations of diseases, and this, in colloquial terms, is tantamount to concluding that "once a dog is dead, its rabies is dead".

Allopathy therefore applies the principle of "opposition", whereby the visible manifestation of a disease is treated with chemical substances that counteract that symptom, which gives us the "*antis-*", antispasmodics, anti-inflammatories, anti-depressives, etc. Confronting this medicine, which we may also call "hegemonic, cosmopolitan or industrial", are other medicines that have gained ground insofar as they have been accepted by official health plans, as is the case of homeopathy (Greek *homo*=equal to, and *phatos*=disease), which implies a type of medicine that aims to combat disease with the use of medication capable of producing in a healthy individual the same symptoms as presented in a sick person. This principle of "similitude" explains how a manifestation of disease is overcome by the presence of a similar manifestation, not by a contrary manifestation, so that the healing of the pathology occurs without the secondary effects that accompany the use of allopathic medication. As regards its conception of disease, the differences are even more evident: homeopathy sees disease as the result of a bio-energetic imbalance affecting the whole organism. Disease, for homeopaths, is not external to the patient but is an internal characteristic of this imbalance, localized at those points indicated by the individual's predisposition. The advocates of this medicine often use a phrase that helps us understand this definition: "One is not sick because one has a disease but one has a disease because one is sick". In other words what is important here is an integral and holistic perception of the human being, which means that disease is merely the visible detonator of a previous asymptomatic condition, an underlying flawor disorder in the individual which only becomes apparent with the disease. In other words, disease, according to this conception, is endogenous to human beings.

In contrast, disease from the point of view of allopathy results from various types of external factors that invade us. Disease is therefore what makes the person sick. This principle is useful to its advocates to insist that "symptoms define diseases". It is a vision according to which disease originates outside the human being, and this implies that we give up in advance on the idea of treating disease at earlier stages. These allopathic viewpoints, for example, attribute disease to environmental factors, and clearly oppose the homeopathic possibility that defines disease from a less invasive perspective or, as we could say colloquially, "to tie up the dog in order to control the rabies".

In any case, where Western faculty medicine is progressively accepting other alternative types of medicine such as radiesthesia, acupuncture and Kirlian photography, we may hope that *healing* based on frequencies of unknown origin may also come to be accepted one day. The example of acupuncture shows how far we still have to go for this acceptance to come about. It was not until Russian scientists were able, some decades ago and with the use of radio-isotopes, to detect the existence of energy channels or conducts in the human organism that we were able to understand how, when these channels were affected by the acupuncture needles, chain reactions were unleashed that were able to cure a broad range of ailments and a number of diseases. Yet it took over 2000 years for this type of alternative medicine to be incorporated in the state health plans of a number of countries.

Other alternative medicines that are increasingly accepted are related to radiesthesia, a particularly useful diagnostic technique that uses pendulums or other such devices to detect energies or even extrasensory information, just as these devices are able to provide credible indications of the presence of water or of mineral veins underground. From Latin *radium*=radiation and Greek *aesthesia*=sensory perception, the word radiesthesia indicates the human organism's ability to respond to radiation from within the earth, a technique that is clearly controversial yet is astoundingly efficient in the detection of certain diseases. Yet again, acceptance has been given to the Bach flower remedies, that use 38 flower essences to treat diseases that, according to its proponents, stem from profound distortions of emotional and mental balance in human beings; they claim that these essences are able to produce states of being that are conducive to healing and improvement in certain types of disease, particularly those whose evolution towards more advanced stages relate to upheavals in levels of stress or anxiety, or where patterns of depression favour somatization with the appearance of particular pathologies.

We live in a time that is unique and critical in that the generalized crisis in health systems, the concerns about synthesis drugs and the automation of medical diagnostic processes have led to an atmosphere allowing alternative medicines to no longer be looked on as scientific heresies. Data of Kirlian photography showing the aura of a finger as different to that of a coin is serious evidence of the presence of energy that is real even if it's origin is probably unknown. To resume, what we should precisely aim at is to approach, without fear or false expectations, an area of medicine which, like *vibrational healing*, can throw light on the existence of particles of possible cosmic origin that are able to help us to overcome disease.

CHAPTER 1

HEALING: TOWARDS A MULTIDIMENTIONAL FORM OF MEDICINE

How should we view the many forms of healing? Are they mystical, supernatural phenomena, belonging to the realm of things that cannot be explained? Or are they, as extrasensory manifestations, able to be explained and tested scientifically in a way that allows us to visualize an as yet undiscovered world of energies, in the form of vibrations present in the universe, that are common to cells and atoms?

If we place healing in either of these perspectives we are faced with a serious problem since clearly it is a concept which, for the vast majority of people, has associations with a broad range of social phenomena including religious perceptions, beliefs, superstitions and every kind of supernatural and unexplainable experiences that come to be confused with extrasensory phenomena, which for their part form a world where scientific explanation is possible.

It is not easy to answer these questions that introduce our reflections on healing, particularly when our aim is to refer to healing as an area of medical practice having immense therapeutic potential but which Western universities of medicine nevertheless still views with mistrust. There are a number of reasons for this, the main one being the semantic problem stemming from the fact that Christian civilization deliberately confuses "healing" with "miracle", a comparison that is particularly unhelpful when we are attempting to investigate scientifically the potential of cosmic vibrational frequencies that, in my view, are able to bring about improvements in the human organism.

This being the case, with the conceptual boundary between extrasensory experience and mystic/religious manifestations being so tenuous, there is little margin for a full understanding of a therapy such as *healing* whichtheorists of medicine insist on including—derisorily—at the residual end of the catalogue of therapies, among other so-called "alternative" medicines.

We are clear, then, that the *healing* we are dealing with in this book has nothing to do with mystic/mythic/religious experiences, nor with the undoubtedly real healing powers of faith. We are dealing with the unexplored world of all that escapes what is tangible to our five senses, and in particular with a form of *healing* which is acknowledged as medical practice by certain highly respected representatives of conventional medicine, i.e. "Western scientific faculty medicine". For our reader's peace of mind, the concept of *healing* about which we will be dealing in this work refers to a therapy of incalculable value for health which, though as yet unknown to many doctors and patients, will in all probability be successfully confirmed by scientific testing though for now we are only able to glimpse that the origin of its therapeutic potential derives from cosmic energies whose existence has been suspected for at least 500 years.

WHAT FORM OF HEALING ARE WE DEALING WITH IN THIS BOOK?

I shall now throw light on the range and dimension we will give in this book to the term "*healing*". The definition I incline towards outlines that "healing should be understood as the sudden, complete and almost total cure of organic damage that takes the form of the repair and/or restoration of the affected tissue and which takes place over a period of less than 24 hours". In short, it refers to a cure, which in most cases is unexpected, whereby a patient successfully overcomes a severe disease.

This being the case, it is essential to explain why *healing* is absolute, sudden and complete. Firstly, it is conceptually clear that being healthy is in itself an absolute: "one is either healthy or one is not". To be healthy is the opposite of being ill, although it seems redundant to say so. And we should look at the aspects of the absolute nature of *healing*, since modern medicine does not necessarily aim to eliminate the causes of illnesses.

We also affirm that *healing*, in addition to its absolute nature, should be sudden and complete, which is to say that we are dealing with tissues that will be fully repaired.

I must stress that my experience of *healing* occurs as a result of a very brief application of energy, produced in any place and at any time, whatever the patient's mood, religious convictions or spiritual attitudes.

But this condition cannot be ignored: *healing* is not a privilege reserved exclusively for believers, whatever their religious faith, and this fact tells us that the curative benefits of *healing* are always within reach of any person wherever they are at any moment of their existence.

There is, however, one requirement on the part of patients without which it is impossible to obtain results. This is the patients' will, based on their clear and genuine desire to overcome the illness; in other words, the subject's desire combined with their action.

If we agree that the patients' will is a pre-condition of my undertaking my therapies, we are forced to consider the case of patients under the age of 12, before which age personal will is not an element that can be taken for granted, as it can be in the case of adult patients.

Yet the answer to this question throws up more light than

shade, precisely because a child's mind is not obstructed by negative thoughts that might block the energies of my therapies. Indeed, young patients come to my sessions with a greater cerebral openness than that of older patients who may have a greater knowledge of the type and dimension of their illness.

Astonishing results can also be obtained with pre-adolescent and adolescent individuals so long as their will is on our side, which highlights the fact that where the subject of treatment has a less contaminated mind and in addition a greater sense of need to get better, then my treatment has a greater chance of success.

In this manner, the patients' response in reversible diseases tends to be successful, even where the diagnosed disease is so serious that itcauses them to have worrying degrees of anxiety. In any case, we need to refer to the limitations I face in my practice of *healing*. These limitations relate particularly to the difficulties involved in treating degenerative diseases and malignant tumors.

On the basis of what we already understand as *healing*, of which we have already spoken, it is important in turn that the reader becomes familiar with what we have decided to designate, in the context of this work, as "astonishing cures". It is essential to define these, not only to distinguish them from *healing* but also to identify the type of disease that can most commonly be overcome with the help of this method.

ASTONISHING CURES

An "astonishing cure", as compared to what is offered by other types of medicine, involves afavourable and outstanding outcome resulting from a whole range of energy healing therapies acting successfully in the space of less than three days.

We are therefore talking about outstandingly effective therapies and procedures, in that they are techniques that provide greater advantages. Among these we can mention the cure of diseases related to arterial-venous insufficiencies of the lower extremities, whereby they are in most cases able to avoid the amputation of legs due to the presence of invasive gangrene and necrosis.

The effectiveness of this type of healing therapy is based, in the case of cardiovascular diseases, on the ability of the organism's vibrational frequencies to liquefy the blood, reduce its viscosity and hinder rapid coagulation, all of which, as we well know, contributes to improved circulation in and oxygenation of the tissues.

It would seem that the red corpuscles undergo a dissociation, which opens a greater field of the surface of the erythrocytes, thus allowing greater oxygenation. Where there is greater agglutination of red corpuscles there is less oxygenation and greater blood viscosity, thus arterial obstruction is more likely, with probable consequences of arterial and coronary thrombosis.

WHAT IS NOT THE HEALING WE ARE DEALING WITH IN THIS BOOK?

We have already seen that *healing*, for us to consider it as such, needs first of all to be absolute, sudden and complete. It follows that where any of these conditions is absent we are dealing with many treatments and procedures offered in most cases by other types of medicine that we would in no sense catalogue as *healings*.

Let us take things one at a time:—in cases of *healing*, patients' recuperation must somehow be spontaneous, involving a rapid and lasting change. For the reader to have a greater understanding, let us say that both these conditions—speed and durability—need to be understood as advantages specific to *healing*, though they are nevertheless relative insofar as it is clear that patients' responses will vary depending on different factors such as age and the complexity of the disease.

Taking into consideration both these concepts—speed and durability—, what is really important about *healing* is that both advantages be manifestly present as compared to treatmentsdelivered by other types of medicine. Indeed, the speed of a patient's response to a healing process is far greater than can be expected of other pharmacological or surgical treatments, which in addition produce collateral effects that damage other organs and tissues.

Durability, understood as the absence and non-recurrence of the targeted disease, is similarly superior to other procedures that exclude *healing*. The successful treatment of certain types of cancer—for example bone cancers, muscular cancers and lymphatic cancers—is viable with my *healing* processes, whether or not they are accompanied by traditional oncological treatments (chemotherapy), except in the case of surgical interventions—as with amputations— and in most cases the results are lasting.

WHERE FIELDS OF MEDICINE MEET

We need to underline the importance, in certain cases, of considering combining my therapeutic process with non-invasive oncological processes as a means of obtaining the best results in the treatment of certain types of cancer. The possibility of achieving this fusion should not be looked upon as a heresy of medical science, since the aim is to exhaust all options in order to avoid those disastrous situations—amputations and/or mutilations— in the struggle with cancer.

Unfortunately, this tragic option is favoured by the majority of legal structures round the world. This final "authoritarian" option seems to be enshrined in the legal codes of most countries, with exceptions where the norms have recently been modified with a view to approach the problem with a broader understanding of oncological pathologies.

In order to create an adequate atmosphere to the integration of important therapeutic treatments of different medicines, able to avoid amputations in the struggle with cancer and other diseases, it is necessary to open a profound debate about the orientation and quality of faculties of medicine throughout the world, based round the fact that their mission is to shape a new professional who is perfectly aware of the pros and cons of therapeutic procedures derived from the different forms of medicine, so that doctors may develop enough judgment to undertake their profession in the best and most objective way, offering patients the best options for their recovery.

The confused framework within which the term healing is used often includes references by many people to non-traditional processes, as for example *reiki*, a type of medicine that is even promoted in the media as part of a varied assortment of esoteric treatments, with the result that ill-informed patients imagine this technique to be synonymous with vibration *healing*.

We shall see further on that in *"reiki"*. The therapist literally imparts to the patient his own energy, thus exhausting himself. Yet this is not the main criticism one may level at *"reiki"*. I base my opinion of this therapy on the scant or non-existent possibility of scientific confirmation that would, for example, make it possible to demonstrate thermographic alterations in volunteer patients at any moment and in any place, which would allow us to identify graphs of the inhibition of germ growth and other alterations in those undergoing this therapy.

Other techniques that can be confused with the type of vibration *healing* that I work with are based on artificial electromagnetic frequencies resulting from the application of magnets and crystals and others achieving thermic alterations with the use of infra-red rays.

I have doubts about therapies now being promoted by certain multinational businesses that use artificial frequencies based on infra-red rays combined with the yadé stone, and my doubts relate to the possible alterations in energy resulting in premature ageing and wear of the cells, since they provoke a change of the electrical potential of the membrane as a result of the modifications in the flow of sodium and potassium which is damaging, possibly irreversibly so, to those membranes or cell filters and, by extension, inhibiting of their potential for action and thereby damaging to the nervous system.

It is in other words plausible, in such cases, to expect premature ageing of cells and a deterioration of the nervous system, which would herald, among many other alterations, an acceleration of diseases such as osteoporosis.

Such electromagnetic currents, which are very commonly used in various therapies that today are very fashionable, in fact produce an artificial and transitory charge of energy which generally exceeds the needs of the cell, thus giving it an "extra dose" of energy which accelerates its deterioration.

This phenomenon occurs, among other reasons, because it is simply impossible to calculate the discharge of electromagnetic current, with the effect that the cells are indiscriminately energized in the course of the therapies.

Of course the patient's response to this type of treatment tends to be positive in a first phase, insofar as the patient experiences a relatively quick improvement which is unfortunately not sustained over time, since the individual's mechanisms of recovery from this physical depletion are slowly reduced.

In other words, though an individual treated with currents and magnets may indeed feel an improvement, we can also affirm that these therapies fail to produce an adequate 'coding ability" in the human organism, with the result that the cell is unable to establish a satisfactory 'memory' of its response to the various stimuli, which all implies failings in this feedback and consequently increased cellular damage.

As a result, those who undergo these therapies begin a slow process of energy loss, because the energy deposits are slowly depleted, and they therefore have to make ever more frequent demands on their reserves.

Despite this fact, therapies based on currents and magnets should be allowed for sports injuries where competitors need urgently to participate in tournaments. In such cases, moderate application of electromagnets is advisable only when the injuries are slight and the treatment includes the prescription of analgesics and anti-inflammatory medicines.

My support for this exception has a logical explanation: high level sporting activities involve excessive use of athletes' joints, so it is acceptable to use a treatment that is as little invasive as possible and is nevertheless efficient, such as magnet therapy.

On the other hand, my opinion is radically opposed to the use of any kind of current in order to stimulate the central nervous system of children suffering from brain damage. I emphatically hold that this mechanism is unsuitable, because in these cases the damage to the brain's cellular membrane is enormous.

In effect, the electric changes cause permanent damage to the balance of this cellular membrane, so the use of electromagnetic beds is inappropriate; not only does it increase the physical damage I have referred to, but the patient's improvement is transitory and these treatments also tend to present a certain addictive tendency.

The reason for this addiction relates to greater energy damage in these patients due to the use of electromagnetism. In brief, we are presented with an unpredictable variation of the electric potentials, which is the undoubted cause of this cellular damage and certain types of cell fatigue that cause the patient to "feel a growing need" for this type of electromagnetic appliances.

The worst consequence of this treatment relates to the fact that the organism becomes incapable of sustaining without assistance its own electrical potentials. As we know, membranes have an electrical potentiality, a determined quantity of micro-volts, which are affected and altered when the organism receives indiscriminate amounts of external physical energies, causing the sodium and potassium balance of the organism to begin to deteriorate. All this is to be observed in the case of electro-stimulation with heavy charges applied to children suffering from cerebral paralysis. In these cases damage is caused to the potential for action carried by the electrical impulses within the nerves, which in turn causes deterioration of the more complex nervous system.

This type of consequence is less serious in the case of ultrasounds, although the Doppler can potentially be a much less harmful and much more efficient way of detecting diseases and anomalies in the human organism.

All the above compels me to insist on the need to find another source of energy that the brain itself is able to codify and assimilate adequately. As we know, our organism has "memory" type cells, i.e. cells "with memory capability"—and this leads us to think that these same cells have the ability to recognize stimuli, among other frequencies.

Brain stimulation aims to produce an auto-regulation at energy level, so that the frequencies are able to set cells in motion as a form of "auto-generator and auto-supplier", without energy losses or distortions that would imply metabolic or immunological damage, as in the case of workers on electricity plants who are more likely to suffer from this type of disorder.

As we know, this type of worker presents with deteriorating health as a result of low level defenses. Despite this, our knowledge about energy levels is still very basic.

It has in fact been a mere 230 years since we have known about energy, and in this time we have uncovered little information about the levels of damage it produces in the human organism. We are far from knowing with any precision the impact on living beings of all the immense traffic of radio-electric and electromagnetic waves, and this includes electromagnetism associated with the habitual use of computers, cell-phones, plasma devices and all kinds of home-electrical goods.

The impact of energy on humans is one of the aspects of science that is least studied. Fortunately, in the field of telecommunications, the subject of electromagnetic contamination is already being discussed. What is certainly true is that today we human beings are over-energized, and this undoubtedly causes deteriorations in human health in a variety of ways.

I believe that the health systems of the world should focus on this matter because, as I again insist, we live today in a world that is contaminated from an energy point of view. There is little awareness of this situation, and in addition, as refers to energy medicine, most of these therapies are practiced by people who are not trained in ideal conditions, so that greater and better efforts are required at this level.

HEALERS AND THEIR PROFILES

Just as we have established the difference between *healing* and astonishing cures, the reader needs to be aware of the similarities and differences between those professionals who deal with the first of these practices as opposed to those who are only able to bring about astonishing cures.

The precise knowledge of the profile that characterizes each of these types of professionals is fundamental when we need to know whom we are dealing with at a crucial moment in our search for health and wellbeing. The difference is also important because of the many interpretations that different cultures give to both terms.

When we look at the English and German world, the Latin root for "healing" is not used since it is associated with the Roman Catholic tradition which restricts the term to the thaumaturgical phenomena of Jesus. In the case of the regions not influenced by Catholicism, the practice of healing during the Middle Ages was the subject of persecutions as it was considered heretical according to Protestant principles.

As regards my therapies, we are dealing with what is known in English as "energy healing", and these should not be confused with miracle healings which are phenomena pertaining more to the realm of faith than to that of medical or therapeutic practice.

For this reason, we wish to reaffirm what we stated earlier on where we defined *healing* as a "sudden, complete and total cure of organic damage", which indicates that my therapy is a procedure that rapidly and lastingly reverses the disease through the application of new energies that definitively replace the old, exhausted energies.

We do not need to deal with the controversies that can be unleashed by my therapies when faced with healing that is not explained by energy regeneration produced by the interferences I am able to produce in the electromagnetic field surrounding the human body. *Healing* here is not to be understood as synonymous with "miracle", i.e. in terms in which the Roman Catholic church uses this category.

Though *healing* can be partially explained in scientific terms, it is not an attribute that any person can achieve, insofar as the application of my therapies requires of the professional who delivers them the fullest conception possible of human existence, which nevertheless implies that when confronting the disease, that professional needs to be aware of all the dimensions of the human being: matter, reason and spirit or, in other words, the physical, the mental and the spiritual aspects.

For the time being it is clear that the human organism somehow gets diseased because of the energy imbalances that result from the somatization of illnesses derived from erratic management of emotions. In this sense, the illness is itself a result of negative emotions experienced by the patient.

It is therefore possible to remove the emotion that causes the illness by "cleansing" the place where the emotion is caused, i.e. the brain, so the use and application of frequencies based on energy vibrations is enough in itself to unleash healing processes that allow the body, like a re-charged battery, to fight successfully against the illness.

Before I deal with the most common practices *healing* professionals use in our therapies it is necessary once again to mention the differences of my work as compared to other techniques of alternative medicine such as *reiki*, a Japanese method aimed at restoring the balance of a patient's physical, mental and spiritual energy, and which involves strengthening that vital energy by means of the transmission of energy from the therapist to the patient.

Concretely, reiki involves helping the patient to overcome some symptoms with energy that the therapist transmits to the patient with whom the therapist synchronizes. This always produces in the therapist an enormous amount of mental, spiritual and physical strain, which no doubt explains why therapists are always exhausted after a session of this therapy.

On the other hand, reiki often fails to produce the desired effects, though it does tend to be effective with rheumatisms and arthritis. However, these improvements are often short lived when compared to the results of *healing*.

"No touch" therapy can be more effective; it was promoted in New York in the '70s by Dr. Dolores Krieger, and she went on to found a school for nursing and medical professionals who were interested in her practice. The method involves applying bio-magnetism to the patient, especially in the case of newborn babies, and this produces a mild sedative effect that in itself is able to cause an improvement in the hematocrits. The development of this technique was possible because Dr. Krieger's work was based on the efforts made by doctors in the United States to emulate the astonishing results obtained by a Hungarian healer who arrived as a refugee after the Russian invasion of his country in the '50s.

Healers, historically and still today, make their reputation for themselves without the need for mediating strategies. As with kings and emperors of old who sought our healings and astonishing cures, today's world sees people willing to seek out and to find healers. We can recall the BBC's programs of the '90s about dozens of healers.

HEALING IN HISTORY

To recreate the history of healing therapies is a complex task entwined in controversies of every kind, and this is due to the great variety of manifestations and techniques used throughout the world. However, just as the names for healing change across the various countries of human kind, healing practices are lost in the very origin of man's obsession: to overcome disease and pain while aiming to live as long as possible, even defying death, if it is necessary.

So the story of healing is not nor can be disconnected from the story of medicine itself. What we know nowadays from the hieroglyphics is that the Egyptians and their doctors were the most acknowledged masters of medical and/or priestly science.

Note that we refer to "medical and/or priestly science", a definition that from the outset places us at the blurred thresholds existing then and still today between the material and the spiritual worlds when we are confronting man's pain in any of its dimensions. When combined in one same profession, both worlds are undoubtedly at the service of that perennial human aspiration to overcome disease.

However, this is not enough to help us understand why particularly the doctors and priests of Egyptian civilization were so esteemed and praised even by the neighbouring kingdoms, which even sent their own princesses in exchange for Egyptian priest/ doctors.

Yet it is a reality that is far from easy for us to credit, that today's scientists would find little or nothing to disagree with when judging the discoveries and methods of these Egyptian priests and doctors for the treatment of a great number of sicknesses.

We know, for example, that they very early on discovered the use of eels producing electric shocks of up to 120 volts in the treatment of cardiac dysrhythmias, and with these they were able to effect cures that avoided the effects of many of the most advanced medicines that are used nowadays with the greatest rigour in order to obtain the best results in the treatment of various heart diseases.

These doctors undoubtedly aimed to improve the quality of life and also to search frantically for ways of prolonging life. Their efforts, given these priorities, even allowed them to perform cranial trepanations without anesthesia, just as the doctors of the Inca civilization of South America did many centuries later.

Healing also appeared in Ancient Greece. At the time of Hippocrates and Plato, in the Fifth and Sixth centuries BC, the celestial bodies seen in the heavens were famous for their healing powers. The Maya and the Aztecs also used advanced medical procedures that are well respected today.

Many centuries ago the spiritual therapeutic practices of tribal Amerindian shamans were well known. In Europe, famous wonder workers were known about in 17th c. Spain. Theophrastus Paracelsus was a famous doctor, alchemist and astrologer in Switzerland and Austria. He was born in 1493 and died in Austria in 1541, aged 48. He chose his name in order to suggest that his healing methods were superior to those of contemporary doctors by referring to Celsus, a 1st c. Roman doctor:— Paracelsus means "equal to Celsus" in Latin.

Paracelsus, who was the first to include minerals in his potions and remedies aimed at healing diseases, is considered a precursor of homeopathy, dedicating the greater part of his life to this science that seeks to combat a disease by means of the same substances that it aims to overcome.

Believing in a "cosmic order" as the last frontier of the material world, this Swiss astronomer considered man to be part of the firmament, so he believed firmly in the essential influence of the stars on the human organism.

Franz Mesmer is a doctor who deserves special mention. He was born in Germany in 1734 and died there in 1815, though most of his medical work was carried out in France because of the political tensions that led to the 1789 revolution.

Like Paracelsus, Mesmer based his scientific work on "the influence of the moon and stars on the human body", and his theories made him a precursor of medical astrology. His investigations included incursions into the field of electromagnetic therapies using magnets with which, in his own words, he managed to produce "artificial tides in his patients".

But Mesmer renounced the use of magnets and inclined towards his theory of animal magnetism according to which healing is possible by means of therapies based on what he called the "ethereal medium", initially a hypothesis concerning a supremely light substance that occupies empty spaces in a liquid form. In fact, Mesmer based his researches on the pre-Socratic theory that held ether to be an element within nature that could be added to earth, fire, air and water. As we know, in Ancient Greece, ether was considered to be a gaseous substance belonging to the world of the gods, and thus different to the air breathed by mortal men.

The medical academies of Europe attempted to discredit Mesmer's work by attacking what he called "magnetic fluid" which he was unable to verify. Had some of the equipment known to us today been available to him then he might have been able to do so. In any case the results he did achieve deserve credit.

Mesmer, considered the father of modern-day hypnosis,

pioneered theories that recognize in some people the ability to cure diseases by means of that animal magnetism, in other words, by probably accumulating energies capable of being transferred to others for whom metals and wood are merely a conduit for these energies.

In short, that Mesmer based the use of metal and wood in his healings was scientifically based on the thesis, proposed in the 18th c., that "the whole universe developed from a homogenous substance, ether, which could later have separated into the millions of elements of which nature is composed".

From this point of view his therapeutic techniques were similar to medical astrology, agreeing indeed as to the reciprocal influence of celestial bodies and living organisms. So the earliest interpretation of this school of medical thought which became so fashionable in the 18th c. held that atoms and cells had a common origin, and it would therefore not be too far fetched to stipulate the existence of an energy contained in them that was common to both.

Of course, in the 20th c., the phenomenon of healing and healers has been documented with greater historical rigour. In Russia, the healing work of Grigori, Yefimovich Rasputin, the infamous Siberian monk, born 1869 and died 1916, is exhaustively documented; he is suspected of treating his patients with intense sessions of hypnotism so histrionic as to have analgesic effects on his distinguished patients, the members of Tzar Nicholas II's family.

Rasputin's healing methods were apparently based on a surprising level of mental domination that he probably camouflaged with disconnected praying shielded by the charismatic and overbearing persona that he adopted after an alleged "vision of the Virgin" that occurred in Verkhoturye monastery. His mysticism intensified after this experience and he joined a sect of flagellants condemned by the Orthodox Russian church. These flagellants sought faith not only through pain but also through sin, which explains their predilection for orgies and drink.

Sai Baba in India, Parvarandareh in Persia and Andalini in Italy, a list of famous healers of the 20th, challenging the material world of medicine with a scientific positivism that held that this material world is not all the knowable to man.

Edson Cavalcante de Queiroz was famous in 1970s and 1980s Brazil. His is a story full of astonishing healings for which he never claimed credit, attributing his powers to the supposed or real spirit of a German doctor named Fritz who had died in WWI and who took over Queiroz's body in what was commonly known as "medium reincorporation", defined as "the transitory possession where one spirit takes over a body other than its own".

Queiroz's renown was so great that North American doctors offered to make him an associate of a famous clinic, but Queiroz declined with the excuse that the spiritual mentor who inhabited him would not allow him to work in that country. Whether true or false, what is really surprising about the story of this Brazilian healer, who was murdered some 20 years ago, is that his feats were published in hundreds of magazines and newspapers. All of them agreed on the effectiveness of his healing methods.

The Catholic Church holds that healing is a gift of God granted only to a few, and has given us a list of healers who in its view were earthly possessors of a divine faculty that transcends their own lives.

This Church believes that the gift of healing is a perfect action of divine, supernatural origin, exercized by God through an individual, whereby famous healers like Padre Pio of Pietrelcina, in Italy in the 20th c., were able to perform astonishing miracles during and after their lives. Padre Pio's special gifts were recognized after his death, and spontaneous (miraculous) healings and cures continue to be attributed to him.

Padre Pio, one of the best-known healers, famous throughout the Catholic world for the stigmata he suffered, was a Capuchin priest born in 1887 in Campania, in the south of Italy, beatified in 1999 and canonized in 2002. He experienced various supernatural powers including bilocation—the ability to be in two places at once—and healing, which he exercised mainly through prayer. He also had extraordinary powers of discernment, particularly in the sense of reading people's minds, a power he used when hearing confessions.

Padre Pio's healing practices, later considered by the Vatican to be authentic miracles which allowed him to be raised to the altars, were exercised from 1940 onwards after he founded the "Home to Relieve Suffering" hospital near Foggia, Italy, which was officially opened 16 years later by pope Pius XII. In this hospital he offered medical and spiritual assistance to thousands of people. This was where Padre Pio combined his gifts of physical healing with an intense spiritual and mystical activity aimed precisely at helping to cure the soul, in the sense that the soul could also help in healing the bodies of the thousands of patients who for many years flocked to the hospital.

The fact that his body remained uncorrupted, added to apparently inexplicable phenomena such as the spontaneous appearance of water and flowers in his tomb, contributed to a persistent sense that Padre Pio's gift outlasted his life. However, there are many in Italy who have ever-increasing doubts about his supernatural faculties. The suspicion that his stigmata were a clever trick has been expressed by many who want to highlight these doubts concerning a figure who awakens both devotion and suspicion among believers and non-believers alike.

We can find further reliable proof of the divine origin of gifts in the case of the German mystic, Therese Neumann, who was born in the Bavarian village of Konnersreuth. She suffered from a rare disease that left her deaf and blind, but made a full recovery in 1923. Three years later, on Good Friday of 1926, she began to experience the stigmata of the crucifixion, and this recurred throughout her life and was usually accompanied by a series of other phenomena including the shedding of tears of blood, the use of a strange language that could—according to some—have been the ancient Aramaic spoken by Christ, and prophesies that often came true.

Witnesses affirmed that, from 1922 onwards, Therese ate no solid food other than the consecrated host, and drank no liquid after 1926. Following her first stigmata, Therese claimed to have "seen" and "felt" Christ's passion during long periods of ecstasy that coincided with the times of the crucifixion.

However, this German peasant mystic awoke little interest in the Catholic Church because, unlike the support that Padre Pio received in Italy during his lifetime, the Pontifical Congregation for the Cause of Saints always maintained that it was impossible to verify proof of her stigmata, her ecstasies and the miraculous cures she worked, and it was not until 2004 that the Vatican declared her a "Servant of God", while the process of her beatification has so far made little progress.

The case of Therese Neumann is not unique in a church which, like the Catholic church, defends the idea that certain people can be gifted by God with supernatural powers or in other words with divine gifts, which has been the case with a number of saints. One of the better known of these was CharbelMakhlouf, a Lebanese ascetic Maronite monk who was born in 1828 and died in 1898 at the age of 70. Following a life of prayer and fasting, and also of preaching and spontaneous healing, he was canonized by pope Paul VI in 1977. His gift of miraculous healing of the sick began during his lifetime but greatly increased after his death. His body remains uncorrupted in his tomb, illuminated by a strange light, and they say a blood-like liquid is often given off, in a case of liquefaction similar to that of St. Januarius in Naples, Italy.

The incorruptibility of some Catholic saints, though some may have been chemically manipulated, is not an obstacle such that we should deny this phenomenon after death. The case of father Charbel in Lebanon is a fact, his body remaining incorrupt for over 60 years, and the same is true of St Bernadette, the child who had the vision of the Virgin Mary in Lourdes, France, in the mid 19th c., and whose body remains incorrupt to this day. A wax mask was placed over her face after many years, but this does not on its own explain the incorruptibility of her body, and this undoubtedly confirms the undeniable existence of forces that make this possible.

The above are clearly "supernatural" phenomena, which have also been seen in other cases such as in the very well known case of St Martin de Porres, who healed so many of the poor and needy of his native Lima, in Peru.

Effectively, though most bodies recognized by the Church as being incorrupt were the product of some biochemical manipulations, it is clear that the incorruptibility of some individuals is a true fact that reveals the presence of supernatural powers.

As we said, the Church's list of healers includes St Martin de Porres, a Peruvian who cured hundreds in Lima in the early years of the XVII c., including some cases considered hopeless, just by the laying on of hands and simple remedies such as placing on his patients a warm cloth or a piece of wood, or other similar procedures which would seem to be innocuous in view of the mortal diseases he fought against over the course of his life.

St Martin was renowned not only on account of his therapeutic abilities but also because he was reputed to have the gift of bilocation; many witnessed to appearances in Mexico, Japan and China, though he never travelled to those countries. Stories circulating in Lima increased the fame of this mulatto saint by claiming that he could levitate while he prayed and could pass through hermetically closed doors. He became so well known that he was visited shortly before his death by the Viceroy, Luis Jerónimo Fernandez de Cabrera y Bobadilla, Count of Chinchón, who kissed his hand and asked him to extend his protection to him from heaven.

But just as human history throws up hundreds of cases of healers, the methods they use can vary considerably. To give one example, Mesmer, the Austrian healer, used a bucket of water while he was healing.

Undoubtedly one of the most extraordinary cases of healing is that of the North American, Olga Worral, a natural healer born in 1906, who decided to make some seeds germinate after they were planted in Pittsburgh, Pensilvania, 1,500 km from her home in New York, to which end she prayed facing towards the seedlings. It was known that she used the power of her mind, working through her hands to the sick people she wanted to cure.

In 1974, Olga's healing powers were subjected to rigorous laboratory testing, including the use of a device, called a cloud chamber, developed by nuclear physicists in order to measure the highest levels of energy particles. The experiment confirmed how Mrs. Worral's hands, unlike those of the researchers, were able to register, on the equipment, waves that change direction as the healer's hands moved around. The frequencies measured by the cloud chamber lasted about 8 minutes before disappearing.

Another experiment in 1974 demonstrated the great capacity of these frequencies to cover huge distances. The waves of energy activated by Mrs. Worral were in effect registered at a distance of over 1.000 km, which allowed the researchers to conclude that her mental action radius was even greater at a considerable distance.

The practical results of this experiment were astonishing. The germs planted in poor soil reacted to Mrs. Worral's frequencies on a scale greater than those that could have been produced by 40.000 earth magnetic fields, the equivalent of 20.000 Gauss. And this was not the end of the proofs, since the scientists applied the same magnetic force to plants in identical beds and obtained energy levels that were 80 times less than the energy produced by the healer. We have to infer from all of this that this woman was probably tapping into a type of energy that was certainly not magnetic.

CHAPTER 2

HEALING IN THE WORLD OF MEDICINE

CONTROVERSIES BETWEEN THE TYPES OF MEDICINE, THEIR APPLICATIONS AND THEIR COMMERCIALIZATION.

At the end of the first decade of the XXI c., the future of Western scientific medicine as a sure and dependable means of treating and preventing illness was challenged by enormous doubts, associated in the main with the collateral risks connected with the majority of traditional therapies.

Along with these criticisms, every kind of seemingly irreconcilable controversies have appeared over the last years between conventional medicine—designated as such because it is probably the type of medicine that is most accepted in political and legal contexts—and the ill-named alternative medicine, understood as "the body of therapeutic practice and procedures used as alternatives or complements to the methods authorized by the health system".

However, the debate is undertaken in such absolute terms that it fails completely to crystallize the scenario envisaged by the World Health Organization (WHO), according to which the XXI c. would be the period when "the different types of medicine would become integrated and would co-exist", a maxim that gives to human knowledge, among others, the main function not only of healing the sick and preventing sickness but also of enhancing the quality of human life.

Unfortunately, this polemic creates an enormous margin of confusion in the public wanting to choose between one or other sphere of medicine, and this leads to an unresolved conceptual issue that includes definitions often dominated by the harmful rejection of one type of medicine by another.

The issue becomes more problematic because of the continuing lack of knowledge as to the differences, within the so-called alternative medicines, between what are purely "diagnostic techniques" and those therapies defined as curative and even preventative, all of which contributes to a dangerous confusion undermining society's faith in medical procedures not financed by national health systems.

What is worse, because of the distance separating the professionals of one type of medicine from those of another—which boils down to an antagonism wherein scientific Western medicine looks down on alternative medicine—it is almost impossible to achieve a political, social, academic, cultural and economic dialogue capable of overcoming the excluding view that each type of medicine has of the others.

Given these considerations it is truly difficult to give *healing* its appropriate place, and this is also in part because healing is a therapy not built on absolute concepts but which understands itself as a practice that, depending on the illness, is able to be alternative, complementary and of course substitutive to both types of medicine: orthodox scientific medicine and so-called alternative medicine. This reflection is important for two reasons: on the one hand, because it allows us to understand that *healing* does not a priori reject either of these medicines nor does it conceive of them as always mutually incompatible; and on the other, because it opens the way to many dimensions in the process of overcoming the illness, since these are not only material dimensions but respond also to the individual's mental and spiritual well-being.

Of course, the fact that healing is open to an understanding with the remaining types of medicine has not yet been met, as it should have been, with openness from most professionals of these schools of medicine, who seem bent on discrediting any advance in medicine that is not based on the application of invasive therapies.

Unfortunately, history is full of cases where conventional medicine refuted and ostracized a series of techniques, theories and procedures that strayed from what had been strictly accepted beforehand. The Hungarian doctor, Ignaz PhilippSemmelweiss, pioneered the fight against puerperal or childbed fever towards the middle of the XIXth c., and his case is symptomatic of how much we still have to learn if we doctors are to overcome our scientific arrogance. It is well known that, in 1845, Semmelweiss discovered that this type of fever, which at the time was responsible for the death in labourof thousands of women, was caused during child-birth by the doctors themselves, who carried the germs of the deadly fever.

Semmelweiss' work in obstetrics, on which he wrote important articles, led him to uphold the thesis that the illness was in fact caused by a lack of rigorously hygienic practice on the part of doctors attending childbirth, so he devoted his life to ensuring that these professionals washed their hands very thoroughly before each birth. However, Semmelweiss' discovery was angrily contested by the gyneco-obstetricians of his day, most of whom doubted his recommendation that student medics attending autopsies during classes of anatomy should wash their hands before entering the maternity wards. Semmelweiss had noted that the death rate among pregnant mothers cared for by mid-wives in another ward next-door was ostensibly lower than in the ward attended by the students of the School of Medicine, which led him to believe thatchildbed fever was caused by bacteria from the corpses used by the students in their anatomical studies.

Semmelweiss died in 1863 from septicemia after deliberately cutting himself with an infected scalpel to prove his thesis. His case is revealing of the degree of reticence that conventional medicine has maintained throughout history when faced with other curative or preventative possibilities in the fight against disease.

In any case, any attempt at placing healing generically and superficially within alternative medicine runs the risk of subjecting it to the theoretical fashions that classify these therapies and techniques as expressions of residual areas of science that are neither entirely serious nor trustworthy nor, indeed, entirely open to proof.

My aim with this book is precisely to attempt to distance *healing* from this interminable debate, and to this purpose I have subjected my therapies to clinical tests that have proved *healing*'s efficacy in the treatment of countless diseases—simultaneously corroborating the absence of negative collateral effects—and at the same time laboratory testing has confirmed how these vibrational frequencies are able, for example, to inhibit the growth of germs and bacteria.

The fact that thousands of patients have sought from me and received successful treatment over the past fifteen years allows me to counter the generic criticism leveled by orthodox medicine against unconventional therapies, to the effect that those responsible for these treatments deliberately avoid laboratory testing of their techniques and procedures.

This, however, is certainly not true in my case. Since the mid 1990s I have focused my abilities on learning and channeling these frequencies as therapeutic instruments, and have been determined to value cooperation with other types of medicine so long as they concurred that the concept of healing was not restricted to curing an organ or a condition in isolation, but sought instead to promote the maximum well-being of patients in their physical, mental and spiritual dimensions. And here I should add some reflections on the long absence of this integral perception of the human being among many of our health professionals, which is reflected in public and private health systems having little commitment to such a holistic view of human existence.

How and where should we place *healing* between the entrenched extremes of conventional and alternative medicine? In order to answer this question we need to pull apart our idea of what is conventional and what is alternative; we need to try to figure out the main differences between those two types of medicine, as also between alternative medicine and those therapeutic methods that are able to replace, or to relieve, conventional medicine.

From a semantic point of view, "conventional" refers to the set of actions that are determined by the canons fixed by tradition or custom. In a broader sense, "conventional" refers to practices that, for the sake of social convenience, are considered to be norms. Which is why it is understandable that the term "conventional" is the most convenient for some authors when referring to Western orthodox or scientific medicine, and the term "faculty medicine" is used by other authors to denote the type of medicine taught in the majority of universities in the world.

Now "alternative" implies that we are able to choose between two or more options, so by definition "alternative medicine" is a valid choice patients can make to combat their sickness, and in no way implies that the procedures of conventional medicine are ineffectual. On the other hand, conventional medicine can be alternative for someone preferring heterodox therapies, but of course we can not deny that nowadays it is accepted that "alternative" medicine is that which avoids the use of synthetic pharmacology and other invasive procedures, which is no basis for claiming that "alternative" refers to categories of less scientific value.

If we use the term "substitutive medicine" we are faced with a similar problem, at least if we hold to the broadest meaning of the term. This definition refers to whatever can replace something or substitute it for something else, though being generally of less quality. This is not the case we are dealing with, but the term "substitute medicine" has become fashionable over recent years in the sense that everything that replaces something else brings with it some new advantages, whatever these may be, particularly as regards the environment. This being the case, the term "substitute medicine" will be useful to identify certain types of therapy that, like *healing*, can offer advantages, as will be seen hereafter, over and above conventional medical treatments, but which imply the certain possibility of causing rapid and stable improvements in patients without recourse, for example, to the antibiotics, analgesics and anti-inflammatory treatments of orthodox medicine.

Finally, "complementary" refers to all that may be needed in order for something to become more complete, and this definition can, in our case, lead us to think that one of the two medicines that we have been dealing with—the conventional and the alternative medicines—has less prestige than the other, or whose role, in other words, though not secondary, is merely complementary, palliative, in the case of chronic or degenerative diseases, or at most, limited to dealing with stress during convalescence.

However that may be, today's citizens are more than willing to accept and to support a combination of medicines, not all of which have legal support, but which can convert alternative into complementary or substituting, or else faculty medicine into complementary medicine, and also any kind of conjugation that allows us as doctors and therapists to benefit from a framework of cooperation able in every case to benefit the patient. And though these citizens have taken this step in the right direction, that is to say they are defending their right to health based on a freer and more mature choice of medicine type, it is we doctors who are called to take this necessary step. The ball is in our court.

Finally, as doctors and patients, what model of medicine should we support? Is it possible to redefine the way medical services are provided round the world so that the interests of patients are promoted over and above the economic interests pursued by the big multinational companies of the pharmaceutical industry?

My opinion is that this scenario could become a reality if two conditions were met: on the one hand, that an open mind be generated among all citizens as regards the fact that we are the sole aim of a public policy that considers health as a priority and key element in the sustainability of development, and on the other, that the provision of medical services should imply a new relationship between the health professional and the patient.

For this dream to be crystallized citizens need to generate enough social pressure to ensure the creation of intergovernmental institutions responsible for worldwide supervision of medicines. At present, this task is merely "entrusted" to the medical authorities of developed countries.

The main thing to highlight is the power of multinational pharmaceutical companies in their relation with national governments, and this means that the situation is even more serious as regards the relation of these companies with developing countries. In the main, the pharmaceutical corporations hold a form of monopoly, because they have almost absolute rights to the production and distribution of medicines.

My concern is not as to whether this power of the pharmaceutical sector is all-embracing, that it covers and includes everything—as I sometimes believe—but to understand why the world's governments still lack multilateral instruments for controlling this industry, which means that we citizens are increasingly worried by the lack of an intergovernmental organism charged with regulating the production, quality, price and side-effects of pharmaceutical products.

Of course, ours is a globalized world, but although the exchange of goods and services is a reality, there are nevertheless many instances where the economic relations between states are regulated, for better or for worse, such as the World Trade Organization (WTO), so it is all the more paradoxical that the health sector lacks international instruments able to exercise efficient, permanent and objective control over the production and export of medicines, particularly when we know that these companies produce a range of substances that, one way or another, affect the whole of humanity.

I would call this a sort of "pharmaceutical colonialism", whereby the major companies of this industry produce not only medicines but also a body of apparently unquestionable scientific literature that allows hundreds of thousands of doctors around the world to promote the medicines via strategic alliances with subsidiary or affiliated companies with considerable power to lobby governments.

This dependent relationship between governments and

multinational pharmaceutical companies is also strengthened by the very absence of multilateral organisms able to verify the efficacy of medicines in the laboratories of the industry itself.

The situation is further complicated by the increasing margin of confusion experienced nowadays between "palliative" and "curative" drugs, which also derives from the over-specialization of medicine, a phenomenon that encourages many health professionals to hold the view that their mission is reduced to "controlling a focal point" of the disease, with no concern for collateral effects, that is, ignoring the treatment of the patient as a whole. In other words, this over-specialization, which may well be justified in the knowledge of human physiology and pathology, focuses the doctor's concern exclusively on one organ or on one area of the body while ignoring the harm that a given medicine can cause the patient's other organs or systems.

All the above implies also that the great majority of medicines in the final analysis are palliative and not curative, which confusion results from the persistence of cultural behaviours prevalent over recent years according to which patients and doctors focus their efforts on medical suppression of pain when this pain is a symptom and not an illness, which means that the drug is palliative and not curative.

Clearly I am not suggesting that the struggle against pain should become a secondary aspect in the old Hippocratic ideal that obliges us, from an ethical point of view, to fight an illness and its manifestations, be they symptomatic or asymptomatic. In fact, fighting pain or the discomfort that accompanies any pathology is and will continue to be one aim of all medical professionals, whatever the type of conventional or alternative therapy they incline towards. What is needed, then, is that the battle against pain be merely part of a war against the illness and not, on the contrary, a situation where the symptoms become the focus of an indiscriminate pharmacological war which in the long term leads to a victory over pain but not over the illness.

This all supposes in practice that, in the twenty-first century, medicine must be open to other possibilities that consider using drugs in a rational and moderate way, without which it will generate, as in the case of antibiotics and a range of other drugs, increased resistances to their curative and also palliative powers, not to mention addictions and dependencies that undermine patients' quality of life. Of course, this call to moderation would be incomplete were we not to consider in depth the contributions that energy healing could offer to conventional medicine, and which allow us to envisage a medical science that is authentically holistic. This outlook offers the best chance of combating the illness from its most remote origin—as would be the aim of an enhanced preventive medicine—to its most extreme consequences, as is the case when we are dealing with chronic or degenerative conditions. And it is in the struggle that governments should support with other therapeutic possibilities complicated pathologies which are probably less invasive and are also able to combat both the symptoms—without affecting other organs or causing systemic damage—and the illness itself and its recurrence.

This cooperation between the different medicines could eventually create the conditions for an authentic curative and not palliative pharmacology, which certainly is not the case today when medicines which are apparently curative cease to be so the instant their collateral effects upset the cost/benefit balance that should guide the world of drug prescription.

Unfortunately there are endless examples of how the interests of the sector's big multinational companies focus their efforts on selling curative drugs that in fact are palliatives. The borderline between the two becomes all the more readily blurred for the simple reason that many patients and doctors tend to confuse the disappearance of the symptom with the disappearance of a supervening illness. In other words, I would say that they underestimate the possibility that a specific illness, even when it is initially overcome with conventional pharmacological management, can eventually give rise to even greater and possibly even catastrophic illnesses. This brings us to the same result: a high probability that many symptoms are therefore taken to be illnesses, which clearly explains the equally high possibility that a patient is prescribed a medication that is only curative in appearance while in reality it is a palliative.

THE PROBLEM OF THE ABUSE OF MEDICINES

Having begun this debate about the continuing margin of confusion between what is palliative and what is curative, I would prefer to think that palliative drugs and therapies should be reserved for illnesses, whether chronic or degenerative, that are definitely incurable, as long as these invasive treatments allow for the alleviation of pain, lower patients' stress, improve their mobility and indeed optimize their quality of life. It is not, of course, a matter of condemning palliative pain management in cases different from these, because as we said before, overcoming pain is a maxim of medical ethics. What I wish to emphasize is that this management can and must be achieved with parameters that avoid putting the patient's other organs at risk, nor any systemic function of the human organism, and this aim can be met if we make provision for a conjunction of types of medicine so that different therapies, including the application of non-magnetic frequencies, may allow for the reduction of the pain and discomfort of an illness while at the same time combating that illness in order to reduce as far as possible the possibility of its recurring and the consequences that it entails.

It is in precisely this case that *healing* therapy can play a fundamental part in obtaining this objective of ending the ever-increasing confusion that health systems and medical teaching have fostered between what is palliative and what is curative, which is a confusion that, in the area of pharmacology, raises the natural suspicion that it is the excesses of world capitalism—a political order in which the big multinational companies have become belligerent actors of the global order—which have led the pharmaceutical corporations to impose all kinds of pressures in order to place their drugs in world markets.

Denunciations of the pharmaceutical industry's voracity are not new, nor are our concerns regarding the indiscriminate prescription of drugs. Voltaire, for example, in the period of the French Enlightenment, had already expressed his concern at the early increase of medication in the eighteenth century, which witnessed a flowering of chemistry within the concert of the natural sciences.

Voltaire's skepticism concerning the excessive use of synthetic drugs resulting from the greater knowledge of herbs that characterized that period led him to give vent to his suspicions that doctors were prescribing "medicines they know little about, for human bodies they know even less about, for the treatment of illnesses they know nothing about". Medicine has, of course, made huge progress since Voltaire's time, allowing us to discover that certain side effects can be guarded against and even avoided, though never to the extent we would wish.

THE PROBLEM OF OVER-MEDICATION IN THE LIGHT OF STATISTICS

At present, statistical data on doctors' abuse of pharmacological prescription can be configured from figures based on those cases where incorrect or excessive medication has led to hospital treatment. According to prestigious periodicals such as Archives of International Medicine, the rate of complications linked to the collateral effects of drug prescription has increased considerably, so much so that the number of serious incidents of this kind more than doubled between 1998 and 2000, while deaths caused by this problem have almost trebled. Thomas Moore, of the Institute for Safe Medication Practices of Pennsylvania, USA, has recently warned that we all need to learn from these experiences in order to guard more effectively against the risks of abusive prescription of medication by health workers. Unfortunately, there are insufficient protections for health system users as regards this problem that is increasing throughout the world.

There are indeed other figures that help us understand the scale of the problem. Moore's team has made in-depth analysis of other information regarding so-called "collateral" damage caused to health and life by the over-prescription of drugs. In the USA alone, the number of deaths recorded by the U.S. Food and Drug Administration grew from 5.519 in 1998 to 15.107 in 2005, while hospitalizations went from 34.966 in 1998 to 89.842 in 2005, which respectively correspond to really alarming increases of almost 270% and 120%.

This increase is the result of an number of factors, one of which is precisely the increase that has been noted in the number of medicines patented world-wide, which has increased by 50% since 1998, which allow one to calculate that the number of complications and deaths due to abusive prescription of drugs is greater than the register of new drugs.

Approximately 15% of the increase seen in the number of complications and deaths due to this problem is related to new substances, including analgesics, whose secondary effects mainly damage the immune system.

The situation could well be even more serious if we take into account the cases that are not reported, so that the real figure of deaths and hospitalizations is much greater. We are unable to measure the gravity of the problem in many parts of the world because detailed studies of the situation are lacking. Daniel Grant, of the Council of the Drugs Commission of the Medical Profession of Germany, referred recently to the scant attention given to the problem when compared to the statistics covering other phenomena, as is the case of deaths in road accidents, which in some countries totals some 5.000 deaths per annum.

In its 2007 report, the German Health Advisory Council calculated that 80.000 patients in Germany that year experienced complications caused by secondary effects of drugs that had been prescribed for them, and that these complications could have been avoided in 40% of these cases.

Unfortunately this is judged to be a growing tendency by the Federal Institute of Medicines and Sanitary Products for Medication, considering that between 1.200 and 1.400 fatalities were the direct result of abuses of pharmacological medication. Ulrich Hagemann is the Director of the Pharmacological Vigilance Department of the

Bundesamt FuerArzneimittel und Medizinprodukte (BaRF), and in his opinion *"these are not the only secondary effects and deaths. We must unfortunately suppose that most doctors do not give information on the adverse cases they deal with"*.

Despite this, my observations and criticisms of indiscriminate pharmacological prescription have nothing to do with *a priori* disqualifications of all that pharmaceutical chemistry has achieved all over the world to benefit humanity, particularly over the last 100 years, though it is true that today we see countless examples of the aggressive way in which multinational companies pursue their commercial aims. Their strategies cover every kind of method: from wide-ranging diffusion of their medical literature which circulates to great effect among health professionals worldwide, to complex lobbying of governments and scientific bodies, including advertising campaigns that in some cases are frankly immoral, in which the companies in the sector openly offer vaccinations and medicines not contemplated in public health plans with the message that their use "will make the difference between life and death".

To this we should add the scant and always qualified information given by laboratories on packaging when referring to the adverse collateral effects of their medicines. These instructions, written in ever smaller-sized print, make no mention of the procedures followed by the laboratory in the elaboration of its drugs, on their secondary effects, or any research by health systems into their effectiveness, if any, or the statistics of recuperation attributed to the drugs or the internal controls undertaken by a given company before the respective patents and/or sanitary registrations were obtained.

Furthermore, what can we say about the non-existent information regarding the origin of the vegetable or animal substance used in the chemical synthesis which give drugs their name, many of which come from regions rich in diversity situated in developing countries and to whose governments they deny any information regarding the commercial use of their bio-diversity.

These reflections necessarily refer us back to the degree of defenselessness that governments, particularly those of developing countries, find themselves in, when they attempt to enforce more efficient controls over imported drugs, over the collateral effects of these on human health, over their pricing and over all kinds of supervisions that should surround the world-wide trade of the pharmaceutical industry.

In addition, we find ourselves faced with a reality of which few users of health systems in the world are aware, and which relates to the undoubted fact that the millions of dollars earned every year by the pharmaceutical industry are in the final analysis contributed by the users themselves, whether they are users at present or potential users of the future, by means of the deductions or salary contributions imposed by law and which are transferred every month to state systems of compulsory social security.

Enriching these companies, which are mainly dominated by European consortiums, eventually places the pharmaceutical industry in a position to consolidate hegemonies in third world countries, which in turn consolidates the overwhelming power of this aggressive industry, one of the most powerful industries in the world.

Contributing users are in effect obliged to invest in the health system a variable but high percentage of their monthly income in order to support the health sector, and these are resources that in theory should cover the treatment of their illnesses throughout their lives. This schema of financing is negatively impacted by the triangular sharing of these resources by the multinational companies, the governments and the state social security system. The most erratic manifestation of this triangulation can be seen precisely in the "commercial circuit" of medicines. We should note the word "commercial" referring to the provisioning, distribution, demand and sale of drugs, a process that obeys the economic logic of capitalism in which the desire for money permeates and dominates the production of substances that relate to none other than the physical and mental health of human beings.

This being the case, and given concerns as to the palliative or curative efficacy of many of the world's medicines and, in most cases, their high cost, health system users are passive subjects of a conventional medication dominated by an almost unchangeable faculty tradition in which doctors, themselves in turn victims of this pharmacological imperialism, prescribe all kinds of drugs whose inclusion in official health plans stem from almost life-long multi-million contracts agreed by governments with the big pharmaceutical laboratories.

Such automation in present day prescription of drugs is the inevitable result of the asymmetrical relation between states and the pharmaceutical corporations, whereby the laboratories of these companies supply, at great cost, the drugs they themselves have pressed on public social health institutions through the intervention of powerful "lobbies", as if they were the only medicines capable of confronting the diseases included in the compulsory health plans. Enormous inventories of drugs in storage facilities or containers are the end result of a trade which, like that of the pharmaceutical sector, is one of the five big industries that move most dollar millions each year around the world.

How, therefore, can doctors, wherever they may be in the world, "defy", if we may use this word, a model of sanitation in which governments establish the list of drugs they may prescribe to their patients? How can these same health professionals confirm the efficacy of a drug or the seriousness of its secondary effects if that government that the health system serves has not been able to verify the production processes of the drugs, their effectiveness, the available statistics on that efficacy and the general map of its collateral effects?

There is not the least possibility at present, as I said before, that governments might find at their disposal an intergovernmental body able to confirm the effectiveness of the drugs that appear on the official list of medicines that patients may hope to obtain from their health systems, thus doctors are wholly powerless in this regard.

I therefore respectfully invite patients and doctors to look closely at the power we have, as citizens contributing the considerable resources that allow governments to pay these multinational companies for all kinds of drugs, despite the fact that there are in place no strategies to avoid, for example, the secondary effects when these are harmful, to reduce the price of treatments replacing them with non-invasive therapies or to develop policies of preventive medicine.

Since we are contributors to the wealth of the laboratories we, patients and doctors, should advocate a strategic alliance that would oblige governments to prioritize health and not to favour the produce of multinational pharmaceutical companies, which in the final analysis seem to impose their own rules when public health policies are drawn up.

The present automation of medical treatments is like a sort of *software* that establishes mechanically for each symptom a corresponding illness and drug, inducing doctors to always prescribe the same medicines. If this automation persist would jeopardize the essence of medicine, which is to view illness and health in a moreoundedway—more holistic to use the philosophical term—and when scientific advances suggest that, in the concept of the world, where the chemical and physical planes are not absolute, and indeed other dimensions, such as those of the so-called alternative medicines, could play a important key part in overcoming illness.

We contributors do in fact, from a certain point of view, hold "all the cards", as the saying goes. This is a fact of which we are not aware, so it is important that as health users we should reflect very carefully on a sphere such as that of pharmacological therapies that affects our organism, sometimes finally and irreversibly, with disastrous consequences to the whole of nature.

There is on the other hand no proportionality between the final cost of drugs and the efficacy that these drugs make claim to on their packaging, and this gives rise to an unusual imbalance, which damages physical wellbeing, as we can see in Europe with the ageing of the population related to the demographic fall, and in addition undermining the confidence that citizens have in the health system that should be less orthodox and more open, as a result, to healing possibilities offered by other types of therapy.

THE ROLE OF HEALTH USERS IN VIEW OF THE HEALTHCARE CRISIS

The active participation of health system users is indispensable if citizens are to become fully aware of the harmful collateral effects of many synthetic drugs, and this would enable demand for alternative medicines to escape their exotic image, where many are confined pejoratively within the naturalist and herbal market where their worth is ranked far lower than it should be, despite the fact that this market is controlled by the health ministries.

Nor is it any coincidence that the vast majority of these drugs are sold without need for a doctor's prescription and are often placed in supermarkets next to soaps and perfumes, as though they constituted a voluntary purchase on the part of users. Of course, the fact that most of these alternative or natural medicines have no collateral effects means not only that they can be sold freely but also, paradoxically, that they are considered by many to be experimental, not serious, and that their exoticism means they have little impact in terms of reducing the price of health, reducing the secondary effects of conventional treatments and optimizing quality so that civil society might include them as wholly valid scientific instruments in the perennial battle against illness.

There are very many examples of patient health failing to improve due to poor drug prescription management. Psychiatry is a clear illustration of this problem, particularly because of the abuse of anti-depressants by many practitioners of this branch of medicine, who increasingly prefer the exclusive diagnosis of a lack of serotonin in their patients' brains to the exclusion of what could be achieved by psychotherapy in a complementary, alternative or substitute way. And incidentally, the criticism of this abuse of drugs in the treatment of mental illness comes from meta-studies by several North American research centrescarried out towards the middle of the past decade.

I believe I am not exaggerating when I state that the indiscriminate prescription of drugs to treat this type of illness is a modern version of the electric shock treatment given to mentally sick patients since the end of the nineteenth century.

In the field of preventative medicine, which in recent years has been reduced to massive campaigns of vaccination, that is to say, assumed exclusively as chemical immunization, we also observe the lobbying power of laboratories to provision state health systems throughout the world with thousands of doses.

When the pharmaceutical industry, despite pressures to include its stocks of vaccinations in government health plans, nevertheless fails in its commercial ventures to sell them off, then their strategy, rather than seeking the prevention of illnesses, is to promote stocks by means of clever and efficient advertising campaigns whereby laboratories sell spurious needs to the population, which in the case of the most vulnerable sectors leads to anguish for the lack of resources to buy the vaccinations.

HEALING: A NECESSARY CONTRIBUTION TO THE WORLD OF MEDICINE

Fortunately there are points of convergence between orthodox and alternative medicine when some doctors recognize the value of certain non-conventional therapies, even though they accept them as alternatives and not as substitutes for their scientific techniques financed by the health system.

However, when doctors of conventional medicine foresee the failure of their treatments, the scientific community does accept non-conventional therapies, though exclusively in an alternative capacity. This occurs where procedures are aimed at treating terminal or chronic conditions, and this acceptance in these cases is likely to be given at the express request of a patient—when it can hardly be denied—rather than from conviction or belief in the alternative therapies.

To clarify this for our readers we need to stress the context of the debate between so-called conventional medicine—that we have also referred to as "classical", 'scientific" or "orthodox", though we do not entirely agree with this nomenclature—and alternative medicine, which for many orthodox doctors is no more than a complementary medicine, if that. But the polemic further intensifies insofar as the best-known definitions of each type of medicine have been phrased pejoratively by their antagonist models of medicine.

Alternative medicine, for its opponents, is a combination of therapies and techniques having no basis in science in that as they are unsupported by quantitative and qualitative verification. This, of course, is an extremist partisan point of view whose purpose is to protect the health sector as the basic model of a hierarchical relationship in which the patient is in adefenseless and subordinate relationship to the health professional.

There is, even here, the possibility that a particular therapy can transition from one type of medicine to another; this occurs when a technique long considered alternative, such as acupuncture, comes to be accepted by conventional medicine. Classical medicine may also exclude an alternative procedure from its protocols of safety and efficiency if it considers its attributes to derive from the so-called "placebo effect", that is to say when an improvement is observed in a patient who has received "innocuous medication"; in this case patients are subjected to a sort of pharmacological simulation able to stimulate the area of the brain which is activated when patients believe they are taking a genuine medicine.

However this may be, the frontiers of alternative medicine have changed over the past decades, leading to a justified critique opposing the view that only those treatments that end up being accepted by conventional medicine are worthy of consideration, and the consequence that all other treatments are judged inferior and unworthy of recognition.

A contrary point of view can also occur among professionals of alternative medicine, in the sense that certain procedures, be they pharmacological or therapeutic, can be accepted and even included in their non-conventional techniques. They do this with the understanding that these techniques are only complementary, palliative or alternative, but never substitutive, except where mediated by respect for a patient's decision to combat the illness simultaneously with every type of medicine, which is often the case as regards terminal and chronic conditions.

As we stated before, the greatest problem facing society today as regards the varied offer of medical attention relates to the persistent confusion that tends to surface when there is a need to find definitions for the alternative therapies. The confusion existing in this domain involves partisans as well as adversaries of one or other type of medicine.

To begin with, and as an example, I should declare that I refuse to accept the term "traditional medicine" as applied to the so-called "western scientific faculty medicine", insofar as the term "traditional" refers to medical practices used by ancestral communities, that is, communities that pre-date the academic and professional categorization of medicine.

To accept without nuance that "traditional" is synonymous with "conventional" leaves in a sort of limbo the ancestral medical practices and knowledge that have allowed many communities to face disease without the collateral risks related to synthetic medicines and, paradoxically, is tantamount to ignoring the contributions that this knowledge has made to the dynamic pharmaceutical industry.

It is useful to analyze the nomenclature we use to define and understand the frontiers between one type of medicine and another if we are to avoid fanaticism and hysteria, and likewise skepticism and fear, in our search for an alternative that human knowledge has provided for us in our struggle against disease and its prevention. This is a tool that is simply there in front of our eyes. It is just a question of using it for our good.

This being the case, the data provided by a former analysis is more than eloquent: Complementary and Alternative Medicine (CAM), has been subjected to semantic manipulations aimed a disfiguring the effectiveness of all the practice exercised under its wing. The acronym CAM is often written sCAM, that is to say, "So-called Alternative Medicine", thus forming the word "scam".

In addition, these same critics believe that where alternative therapies prove their efficacy in clinical trials they automatically cease to be alternative and become part of the patrimony of conventional medicines, thus once more excluding the other alternative treatments.

Many conventional therapies rely on indiscriminate administration of drugs, and the "efficacy" they claim for themselves implies that alternative medicines are all those that can not be proved scientifically. This only confirms the conceptual abyss between all types of medicine, and the lack of desire to seek understanding between them, even though this aspiration is proclaimed categorically by the World Health Organization (WHO).

What is truly important, outside of these controversies, is the increasing degree of recognition that alternative medicine is beginning to awaken in our society, particularly in developed countries. This is noteworthy when we consider that for many decades alternative therapies were held to be an under-developed product of the health sector of poor countries. On the contrary, alternative therapies seem nowadays to have greater penetration in the industrialized countries, where the big multinational pharmaceutical industries originate.

A study produced in 2004 by the National Center of Complementary and Alternative Medicine established, for example, that two years earlier, in 2002, 36% of Americans had used alternative therapies in the previous twelve months, including yoga, meditation, herbal treatments and the Atkins diet. This same study indicated that if healing was included in the list, the figure rose to 62%. Similar studies revealed that, in 1998, 20% of the adult population of the United Kingdom had used alternative medicine in the previous twelve months.

The reason for this confidence, that continues to grow despite the lack of legal support for these kinds of medicine, is due to growing awareness of the negative collateral effects of drugs and the no less traumatic consequences of amputations and/or organ removals, among other surgical interventions.

HEALING: AN ALTERNATIVE TO SURGERY?

From a historical point of view it is no exaggeration to suggest, for example, that surgical interventions will in the future be as obsolete as certain medieval medical procedures and diagnoses appear to us today, such as when dementia and other mental imbalances were associated with the notion of "the primacy of malign spiritual possession".

On that score it is worth mentioning now something which may be an advance in the field of surgical interventions. I refer to the practice of surgery without anesthesia, which is a meeting point—and a point of agreement—between conventional medicine and practices that avoid drugs such as the powerful sedatives used by anesthesiologists. I should in fact mention that my incursion into the world of healing began with my experiences in the practice of surgery without anesthesia when I discovered, in the early 1990s, that I was able to induce states of sedation deep enough to allow for certain types of surgical interventions.

The surgery without anesthesia based on the states of sedation I induce in my patients differs from hypnosis, which is a technique whereby the patient is conscious throughout, this having a therapeutic function insofar as it allows for feedback from the patient that can later be used in psychotherapy.

This difference is essential in order to understand why I need to induce in my patients a much deeper trance, so that they are unconscious long enough for surgery to be carried out for as long as is necessary. The types of operation that are possible without anesthesia with my procedure include leg surgeries.

Performing surgery without anesthesia was of course only the beginning of a broader practice, from which I observed that my therapy had the additional effect of healing patients suffering from pathologies other than those requiring my surgical interventions, or additional to the procedures I undertook in the therapeutic rehabilitation of children with brain damage.

Effectively, it was when I needed to overcome many clinical profiles that were unlike those of most people who came to me for treatment that I began to make important discoveries. I associated these with the magnetic fields I was working with at the time, in other words, I mistakenly assumed that my energy was a type of electro-magnetism, but later on I rejected this probability when I was able to compare extensively my work with therapies used by countless professionals of bio-energetic medicine.

I was able to collate and compare the results of my therapy with therapies—based on magnets and electrical currents—that were common to bio-energetic medicine in the 1990s. This task confirmed my confidence in my healing powers and I began to realize that these powers were not of a magnetic type.

My energy was achieving therapeutic results far superior to those achieved by bio-energetic medicine, so I concentrated on the idea that I was dealing with a magnetic field that contained no magnetism, or with a kind of magnetism that was unlike any we knew about.

HEALING AND THE LEGAL LIMBO

I suspected that the therapeutic properties of non-magnetic energies were far superior, and this suspicion strengthened as I saw people improving more quickly and achieving longer-term levels of healing. Indeed, in some cases they achieved levels of healing that seemed impossible, and all of this of course ended up leaving a deep impression on the families and friends of those I treated at that time.

Praise I received for my work with these patients, and the results themselves, encouraged me—with the support of laboratory experimentation— to continue investigating the quantitative and qualitative level of efficiency of my therapy as compared with that of professionals working with bio-energy. These in fact, in addition to a type of conventional magnetism, were offering a series of alternative techniques including homeopathy and auriculotherapy, and also used quartz crystals, geometric figures and colours, indeed a whole range of tools that were complementary among themselves, with the aim of achieving improvements that in any case turned out to be more transitory than lasting.

This being the case, it was no easy task to work with healing therapies during the explosion of alternative medicines that occurred in the early 1990s, so I decided that I would take a sideways step, leaving out my title and pursuing my therapist's work directly as such, that is to say, as a healer now gifted with certain special faculties that have allowed me to combat that range of diseases that I have spoken of in previous chapters.

Obviously, my work as a therapist belongs to a legal context that is favoured by a fact that is certainly paradoxical:—no country has prohibited non-invasive therapeutic practices, that is to say, practices, such as *healing*, that avoid any intervention of the therapist on the patient, whereby the healing professional avoids the use of needles, avoids prescribing medication, avoids even touching the patient during the therapeutic session. I wish to stress that touching a person during a consultation is already somewhat invasive, as is prescribing a medicine or using instruments.

This illustrates how, as regards healing, we are in a legal limbo, not only in the contexts where I have worked but throughout the world. This is the case because of the difficulty of imposing rules that exhaustively prohibit this kind of therapeutic work, and that this type of work occupies a diffuse space that includes aspects that are not only physical but also mental and spiritual.

A patient's right to health and to life is indeed not only a legal right, it also takes a diversity of forms that, in addition to Western scientific medicine, include the legitimate option that is each individual's personal choice, where patients are guided by their own beliefs, which is an area protected constitutionally in all democracies subject to principles that guarantee the right to intimacy, to the free development of the personality, to freedom of religion and to all kinds of cultural rights established for ethnic minorities, as is the case for the indigenous communities of Latin America.

That the law should prohibit these types of therapy, which include healing among them, seems to me to be frankly incoherent in a democratic society, because it implies, as I understand it, a constraint on our rights as individuals to seek our physical, mental and spiritual improvement by whatever means we deem appropriate.

One case that is symptomatic of the enormous questions that are still to be resolvedbetween conventional medicine and healing therapies is that of the German healer Bruno Groening, who was born in 1906 and died in Paris at the age of fifty-three. Groening was famous in the post-war period for his extraordinary ability to heal incurable patients, yet he was a permanent victim of a tenacious campaign to discredit him that was waged by the European medical bodies, despite the fact that they were able to witness truly miraculous cures that he achieved throughout his life, even including the full recuperation of patients with disabilities.

Groening recurrently attributed his healing powers to the existence of a superior energy from which life originated. His story was that of a man who today, fifty years after his death, is an example of how the prejudiced andunderhand attacks of the conventional medical establishment against all other healing options do nothing to favour patients' health and life improvements.

This being the case, the rigid, schematic, radical, dogmatic, conservative and traditional point of view of health systems around the world presents an obstacle favoured bynarrow-mindedness, while only open mindedness will allow us to give enough leeway to people's free will in the search for their opportunities for healing.

The challenge also implies working towards considerable reforms within universities in the field of health sciences, to allow for an opening in faculties of medicine, after 1.200 years of tradition, towards a sort of scientific ecumenism that would allow them to enrich themselves with other concepts, other visions and healing experiences other than those that posit the intervention of physical and chemical elements in the diseased organism as an absolute and thus unchallengeable good.

THE IMPACT ON HEALING OF AMERICAN CULTURAL DIVERSITY AND EUROPEAN PRAGMATISM

That health systems around the world should exclude a priori any option other than the invasive procedures they defend and promote is a fact that also consolidates within a vicious circle the growing costs of financing and sustaining health care throughout the world.

The invasive emphasis of the cures favoured by conventional, traditional medicine, corresponds to the restricted historical frame within which health systems conceive of health and sickness, a frame that is even more inflexible and rigid, and for this same reason is obsolete in those developed countries where most multinational companies of the pharmaceutical industry are based.

This is nothing new, and although the citizens of these countries are increasingly involved in the debate, yet in so-called first world nations, patients and their families continue to be victims of an implacable moralism that conspires against this purpose, precisely when efforts are being made to defend this right by means of non-invasive techniques that are neither pharmacological nor surgical nor of any other kind.

I am far from wanting to engage in unnecessary and inopportune controversies with conventional medicine, particularly when I have shown that I respect the substitutive, alternative or complementary nature allowed in some of its procedures. However, I believe I have the duty to point out the need for a more fruitful cooperation between the different types of medicine, an understanding able to make holistic, lasting and rapid healing of patients into an idea and an aim that can overcome resistances of all kinds, from those linked to professional jealousies between exponents of each type of medicine, to the socio-economic resistances where the rights of patients take precedence over those of pharmaceutical companies.

My experience tells me that, despite the imperfections of its health systems, Latin America is perhaps a region with a society somewhat more open than others to the type of work I have been doing over the last twenty years. This is an advantage for those wishing to advance the immense and unexplored healing potential offered by vibration frequencies.

CHAPTER 3

MY THEORY CONCERNING THIS THERAPEUTIC PRACTICE

What scientific explanation can we give for this *healing* procedure, whose efficacy we have demonstrated to satisfaction? From my medical perspective I can vouch that the therapy I apply has a sufficient capacity of cerebral incidence for a reason that is more physical than anything else:—the brain is composed mostly of water, which clearly is an incomparable conductor.

This being the case, frequencies passing through the hands mean that these frequencies adapt to the brain as they are perceived by the human organism, which results in stimulation of the bio-chemical and immunological mechanisms which in turn activate the central metabolism.

Following this phase, the physical and chemical balance thus achieved re-enforces the catalyzers that we know commonly as enzymes, since all this derives from an astounding recuperation of the immunological mechanisms, nature's tools which, as we know, are the foundation for recuperation in the damaged tissues of an organism.

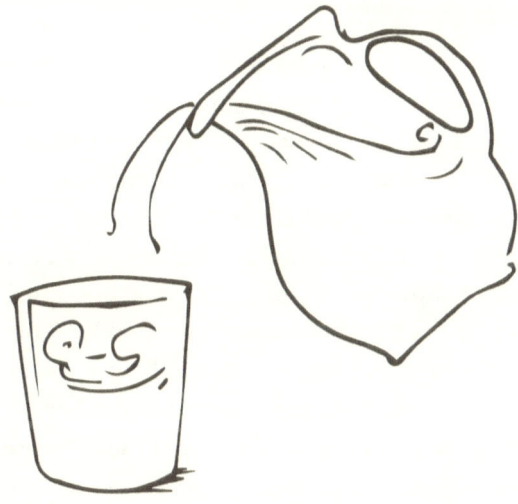

Now all these changes can be monitored scientifically by registering the variations that succeed each other in the temperature of the brain and which are perfectly revealed by the "thermographic camera", and this proof has made it possible to establish valid parameters allowing us to conclude that this partial increase in temperature brought about by the irradiation of energy coming from the therapist's hands causes relative dehydration in the brain, with the result that the patient feels thirsty and needs to take on water.

Naturally, this loss of liquids needs to be compensated by the taking on of water for as long as is necessary, even beyond the period of time during which the patient feels this sensation of constant thirst. Patients often have headache or unease in other areas of the body after the first two therapies, these being secondary effects of the therapy and being counteracted with an increase in consumption of liquids.

According to my theory, this leads to an initial imbalance in the bio-chemical mechanisms, such as gluconeogenesis and subsequent increases of lactic acid in the tissues, for example. In most cases, decompensation is also caused by the natural effect of elimination within the organism and because of this procedure, of excessive toxic substances within the cells.

Gluconeogenesis is a fundamental intracellular metabolic mechanism whose important function is to control glucose throughout its distribution as it is converted to fructose, which is far less harmful to the organism. Lactic acid is produced in this process, as waste product derived from this transformation and distribution process, and this lactic acid is deposited in the cells and causes unease and pain, such as cramps for marathon runners when the process occurs too quickly. From a chemical pint of view, gluconeogenesis requires the use of various amino-acids such as lactate, pyruvate, glycerol and other substances. All amino-acids except leucine and lycine are able to provide carbon for synthesizing glucose.

As we know, the accumulation of substances always results from years of consumption of medicines on the part of patients who eventually store in their organism so much toxicity that it can only be drained away by increased hydration. For some patients there is a true "energetic shake-up", which in its most extreme form can last from three to six weeks or even more, though I find that this collateral effect is positive insofar as I consider that the patients being treated are immersed in the first phase of their recuperation, which is always stimulating for my daily work as a *healing* therapist.

Now we need to delve further into considerations of a scientific nature in order to demonstrate the efficacy of my therapies beyond the period of time strictly required for the *healing* procedure. I refer to an aspect that fundamentally differentiates my therapy from other alternative medical therapies, where the healing effect on specific symptoms of illnesses lasts as long as the respective consultation or therapeutic practice.

In other words, it is clear that in these cases we are dealing with the absence of one of the characteristics that in themselves define the healing: that is the durability of the cure, where this duration is continuing for a longer period than the treatment itself, which allows for a reduction in the margins of recurrence of the illnesses that the *healing* therapies are combating.

Thermic and energetic changes at cerebral and/or global levels are shown by the thermographic camera to be induced by the frequencies I work with, and according to my theory, the bio-chemical stimulus produced by the changes in temperature are reflected in sustained processes of dehydration

In my opinion, the persistence of thirst even after treatment has ended is a further proof of activation in the brain itself of processes of auto-regeneration of frequencies. The existence of this type of "frequency generating motor" most probably explains the lasting character of the recuperation of the tissues of the affected human organism.

The question we now need to ask ourselves relates to why the bio-chemistry of the brain is activated, this being, on the other hand, an organ that controls the fundamental functions of human existence in its fullest and most holistic dimension, which even involves—and why not?—the condition that makes of man a spiritual being.

The answer to this question poses an enigma for science. Would it be possible to speak of a frequency codification? Are we dealing with a phenomenon where, as with hertz waves, the frequencies underlying healing therapy are subject to emission/reception processes?

If this is the case, my therapy is at a stage where the emission of frequencies does not imply that these are transferred to the patient— as occurs with reiki—but supposes their activation—or auto-generation of frequencies in patients' brains—due to stimulation from the frequency emission that codifies the receptor.

The challenge is precisely to involve scientific knowledge as a whole—and not only that of medicine—in the task of responding adequately to the question of why this auto-generation of frequencies in patients' brains occurs.

For now, what is fully accepted is that *healing* therapies have a measurable secondary effect or external manifestation—i.e. the changes in brain temperature—and also an undeniable healing effect. The way forward at present is to discover the origin of these unknown frequencies, which could undoubtedly be key elements in the scientific advancement of medicine in the future.

In previous chapters we have explained the minimum characteristics and conditions that define both healing and healers. We have also said that *healing* is not the gift of those believing or practicing a particular religious confession.

We should nevertheless ask ourselves, at this stage, what type of patient and what pathological profiles are likely to make a *healing* therapy more effective. To my mind there is no clear model of the type of patient who is technically more inclined to be effectively treated by my therapy.

This point is also demonstrated by the fact that my therapy is usually addressed more to groups than to individuals, which suggests that it is difficult, if not impossible, to know which patient has that profile that can supposedly be considered more favourable for the success of the healing process. My conclusion is not simply an a priori judgment. For years I have tried to discern that profile that would be able to give me guidelines for knowing what people and diseases I have to deal with on a daily basis. And it is undoubtedly in this quest that health professionals could fall into dangerous out of date and obsolete positions that would liken us to those monotonous hierarchical doctor/patient relationships of Western scientific faculty medicine.

However, in this search for the right patient I have certainly met with more than one surprise. Indeed, I have many times come across situations in which I have spontaneously discovered that the energy "works on its own and in its own way", and "chooses how" it adapts to an organism in order to cure it, or in other words, the organism readies itself at a given moment to receive that energy. Whatever the case, we know scientifically that "energy is information, and as such it travels".

This situation sometimes strikes me as so astounding and unpredictable that I often assume a priori that my treatment may not be very successful in the case of certain patients. In such cases I often feel at the outset that nothing positive will probably happen during and after the therapy, yet the patient's response gainsays my doubts once I discover that the disease has been turned round and that the patient is on the road to a recovery that I had not expected.

In these situations I have to deduce that we are faced with a type of frequencies of which we know little, yet which carry specific information—of a cellular or metabolic nature—which is able to fit into the organism in order to strengthen the immune system.

I tend to think, on this point, that such frequencies may include not only material dimensions—able to be confirmed in the laboratory through the bactericide effects of my therapy—but also mental and spiritual dimensions, which we could associate to the conclusions of anatomical studies in the United States which have concluded that there is a "spiritual centre in each of us". It may then be that human beings, on the basis of this spirituality, are able to establish links— via frequencies—between all these dimensions, in order to achieve practical effects with the healing of diseases.

There are varieties of healers, and there are likewise varieties in the practice of healing depending on the methods used. In my own case, the practice of *healing* requires no great effort of concentration aimed at activating thoughts towards the homogenization of energies, in order for these to achieve the necessary balance. This balance brings about a change in the energies of the patients when I approach them and make short passes over them with my hands.

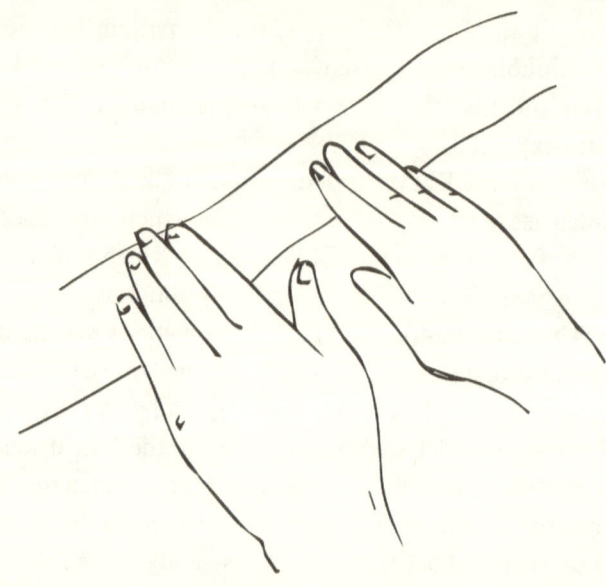

Since I am generally dealing with group therapy, the action I take in each cubicle with each patient is to bring my hands close to the head or to the affected part for a few seconds, always at a minimum distance.

I must mention, the better to explain the procedure, that when I execute these hand movements I do not concentrate specifically on the type of illness of each patient, so in certain cases it becomes necessary to bring my hands close to those damaged parts of the organism which are the focus of the therapy.

SCIENTIFIC PROOF

Surprising results were produced by laboratory research carried out in the 1990s when comparing bacteria treated with synthetic drugs—essentially antibiotics—with bacteria treated with my energy therapies, where I used my hands to transmit energy vibrations. They proved that my energy treatments were as effective as the antibiotics in destroying certain bacteria that previously had only been treated with "dangerous" drugs, bacteria we know to be ever more resistant to an increasing number of those drugs. The path leading to this demonstration began in 1995, when we decided to undertake a series of studies on the inhibition of germs in the laboratory of Facatativá hospital. The experiments were supported by a select group of bacteriologists and doctors from that institution, and the end result of our observations was an astonishing level of growth inhibition in streptococcal and staphylococcal bacteria and in a fungal infection known as moniliasis.

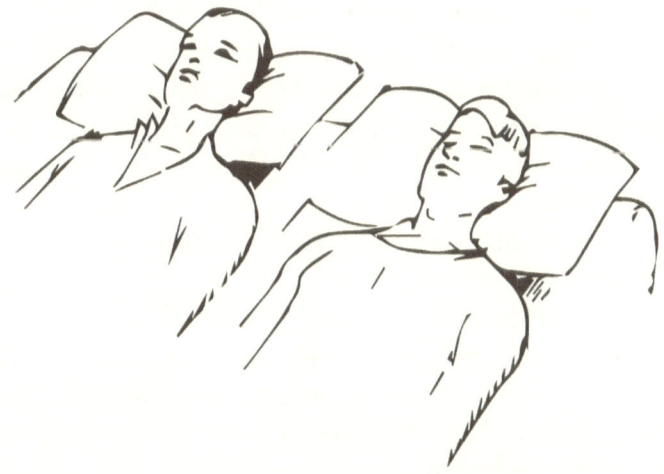

The experiment consisted in applying energy via my hands to a culture of bacteria and fungi for approximately ten minutes and from a distance of one inch above the laboratory dishes, after which the culture was checked every 12, 24 and 48 hours. At the end of this period, we were surprised to discover that growth had been inhibited, in some cases, by 90%! The conclusion was that under conditions established by the WHO, this in vitro procedure had achieved better results than those achieved with antibiotics, which in other words meant that the therapy definitely was effective as a bactericide, and was therefore capable of destroying microorganisms causing conditions such as dermatitis, tonsillitis and erysipelas, among others.

The therapy not only proved its efficacy as regards the bactericidal aim I have described, which I have no doubt in attributing to the frequencies, but in addition the therapeutic practice had proven effects as regards "immunomodulation", which we understand as the relaxation experienced by patients, reaching almost trance-like states, which achieved something that was very important for their recuperation, i.e. a sustained increase in their immunological level that warded off the possibility of the condition recurring.

Immunomodulation, with its sedative and tranquillizing characteristics, allows for successful stimulation of the central nervous systemand this in turn produces feedback that guarantees a stable and sustained improvement in the patients' immunological systems, this being part of my therapeutic method. The father of immunomodulation is Dr. Howard Hall of the Children's Hospital of Chicago, who in the 1980s carried out serious and exhaustive studies with countless people, particularly students, on the various forms of relaxation management in human beings, with surprising results as regards immunological responses in general. Dr. Hall's contributions figured in various publications, and were particularly highlighted in Neuroscience magazine in the early 1990s. After that experience, that I have no hesitation in qualifying as successful, it would have been worthwhile to have had at that time more support from the health authorities in order to continue the studies, which we wanted to repeat on a larger scale later in Bogotá, in the Nueva Granada Military Hospital.

The bactericidal effects of my therapies, which as I have said are based on the use of my hands, whether or not I establish physical contact with the patient—or with the in vitro culture of bacteria— allowed me to increase my confidence in the enormous possibilities offered today by vibration healings, insofar as the emission of energy necessarily reaches a "receptor or subject" whose own energies are changed, this being manifested mainly through surprising changes in body temperature.

When I work with the electrical potential of bacteria, that is, when I act on bacteria with my energies, the results are astounding yet they have a logical scientific foundation: "the vibration energies act on the intra-cellular metabolism of the organism unleashing chain reactions in the immunological systems and, in the case of infectious diseases, making it possible to combat them more quickly than is possible with antibiotics".

During the 1990s I worked on the therapeutic rehabilitation of children with brain damage in La Misericordia Hospital, in Bogotá, and it was during this period that I came to suspect more and more that energy healing is a technique that is potentially superior to those known beforehand.

The hospital occupies old republican buildings dating from the early twentieth century and has enormous problems that relate to an increasing demand for health services from children with brain damage, and their clinical profiles, caused either by this type of damage or by additional illnesses, improved substantially with my vibration techniques applied to the brain.

The brain, like the operating system of a computer, controls all the functions of the organism, so we can claim that any irrigation of energy aimed at compensating for a deficit, that is equally a deficit in energy, will give to the cells of the brain the strength they need to mend the deteriorated immunological profiles with which human nature is provided in order to combat, on its own, every kind of immunological imbalances that are the principal causes of diseases.

It was then, with no connection to any effort to provide healing with a nomenclature within the changing classification that today confronts conventional medicines with the so-called alternative medicines, that I become even more convinced that *healing* corresponds to a therapy that should eschew the endless polemic between those who consider the two philosophies to be irreconcilable.

I am referring to the controversy whereby at the core of the debate is conventional medicine, which we understand as that Western medicine that views the treatment of illness as a perennial struggle in the material world between the external manifestation of the illness and synthetic drugs or invasive procedures such as surgical interventions which are held to be the only tools capable of halting infections, pain and/or any other external manifestations of the illness.

This polemic likewise advances critiques, some of them valid, of the efficacy of the most common procedures of so-called alternative medicine(though it is my opinion that it is wrongly called alternative insofar as this seems to limit it to a secondary, a last chance, a not too serious character) whose aim is to combat not only the symptoms but also the causes of illnesses, employing for this purpose a broad range of therapies and techniques, many of which even use the "placebo effect" which is defined as "the effect produced in certain cerebral functions by drugs that are chemically innocuous", thus attacking what could be called the "mental source" of many symptomatologies.

Today, proving the levels of efficacy of the different medical procedures is faced with new complications. There is a growing environmental awareness that prohibits the use of primates in scientific experimentation, and to this is added the fact that people are reluctant to volunteer for clinical tests to check the efficacy of drugs or treatments, so that such tests are now conducted with more sophisticated technologies.

The results of laboratory tests on my energy therapies convinced me that this new area of medicine is able to replace even the most orthodox and widely used methods of conventional faculty medicine. The reasons for this thrilling possibility are more than eloquent, insofar, for example, as my techniques can be successfully repeated at any time, in any place and with any patient, because one of the signal advantages of my therapy is that it creates no resistance in the organism, thus eliminating, in other words, one of the main problems encountered by modern medicine, which is the increasingly innocuous impact, according to the WHO, of the antibiotics that doctors prescribe indiscriminately.

Statistics also support non-invasive procedures, whether they be pharmacological or surgical. In the USA, in only the five years between 2002 and 2007, appointments for conventional medicine dropped from 75% to 65%, while appointments for alternative medicine rose from 28% to 35% for the same period, and this reveals a growing mistrust for pharmacological procedures among Americans, despite the fact that their society has legislation that continues to favour conventional medicine.

My therapies also respond to a valid concern on the part of patients regarding the quality of the cures, specifically their lasting effect and the non recurrence of the illness, and this concern places us in the realm of the hippocratic genesis of medicine, which is not the alleviation of pain—which has been and will continue to be a basic aim—but the elimination of the causes of this pain, the prevention of the illness and even the improvement of the physical and mental potential of a healthy human organism.

In order to address this issue we need to focus on a profound difference in the way the professionals of one or other of these types of medicine conceive of illness. It is important to remember, in this respect, a basic principle that is largely ignored by the majority of doctors, that "we are dealing with ill people, more than with illnesses"; in other words we are dealing with people with symptoms, and these symptoms may be the same in different people yet have different causes, be they genetic, endocrinal, nutritional, etc., so we are faced with very different causes, manifestations and consequences of illnesses, and we find that in the long term the conventional invasive, general and indiscriminate treatment brings with it more problems than solutions.

Given that the brain also needs to adapt to the energies transmitted to the patient by the energy healing professional, it is also natural that we are faced with a problem of tolerance to that very energy which makes the healing possible. This, however, is a temporary situation during the first stage of treatment where, paradoxically, the patient presents an increase in sensitivity to pain, due to the fact that the brain is adjusting to the energy inputs that will combat the illness.

While the brain is needing to adapt to the energy, the human body then assimilates the bio-chemical alterations that will be able to activate the production of enzymes in order to achieve an adequate immunological response.

WHAT I REQUIRE OF THE PATIENT

As I mentioned before, I mainly use a group procedure, since I treat 20 to 25 patients simultaneously, who remain on hospital beds throughout the 45 minutes of each therapy. Once I am satisfied that my patients are fully relaxed I go round the room to the beds and approach my hands to the head of each patient for about 45 seconds.

The process is repeated after a recess of 15 minutes. I believe this to be a necessary reinforcement to guarantee the efficacy of the therapy. In certain cases, and depending on the seriousness of the health problem we are dealing with, the patient can request a third nearing of hands for a further 45 seconds. The irregular number of times I go to each bed often gives rise to cordial comments from my patients, most of whom express some anxiety because they imagine their improvement depends on the number of times I spend with each of them. These are almost subconscious complaints.

My answer to these anxious patients allows them to understand that there is no direct relation between one thing and the other; or indeed, they understand that from my point of view the second passing of hands is sufficient for that session, and there is therefore no risk that the patient's organism has not received enough of the vibration frequencies that are the basis of my therapy. Such comments nevertheless do sometimes indicate that for a given patient, the concentration of frequencies has not been as successful as we had intended.

The level of relaxation is therefore essential for the best results to be obtained from the therapy in the least number of sessions. When relaxation is deep it often triggers patterns of sleep during which the application of the therapy can advance more smoothly.

Anxiety management is therefore an important aspect to bear in mind when someone decides to undertake this type of treatment, for my experience tells me that the patient's successful response to the therapy depends partly on a low level of mental contamination when the person comes to the consultation. If we are dealing with anxious patients who have obsessive thoughts it is clear that their ability to concentrate is diminished, though this does not mean that it is not possible to do something else so that this type of person should respond to the treatment.

The above is valid for adult patients. It is worth asking ourselves how much cooperation we can expect to get from children whose desire for recuperation does not belong to a mental state that we can manage before or during treatment. How can we succeed when dealing with one- or two-year-olds whose concentration is practically nil because they lack the ability to reason?

Despite this, and contrary to what one would think, children are more inclined than we imagine as regards obtaining good results from the therapies. The main reason why better results are obtained from this sector of the population suggests, precisely, that the child's mind is less predisposed than that of adults, and therefore offers less resistance to the therapeutic effects of the *healing*. On the other hand, the lack of obstructive prejudices about the treatment itself becomes a valuable ally for the success of the therapy in the case of children between the ages of 7 and 12, as also with pre-adolescents, since their levels of concentration improve as they grow older, this being part of the apprenticeship specific to this age range.

To conclude, as I mentioned earlier, if we need to define a patient profile that provides a good fit for a healing therapy, I would say that such a prototype does not exist as such. For sure, it requires certain conditions that any patient can provide for the success of the treatment, and this contribution is no more than to engage with the therapy with the least possible degree of alteration in their emotional, mental and spiritual state.

On the other hand, my patients claim from their experience to sense the application of the frequencies in very different ways. For sure, they all agree in warning that "it is impossible to define exactly with words" the sensation felt during and at the end of each session.

They admit that it is an unknown sensation, and that it is clear that most of them feel strange.

This sensation of strangeness makes many people come faithfully to appointments with me whether or not they believe in the treatment, for the simple fact of experiencing a sensation that is totally different as compared to the other procedures and experiences of the wrongly labeled alternative medicines.

When talking to some of my patients, they also say they experience different types of numbness, involuntary gastric movements, uncontrollable vibration in their eyelids, the presence of needles moving in circular or linear motion, mild nausea or tiredness. Others, on the other hand, perceive a sort of "unknown power". When they make these statements I observe them and listen, always with an undisguised smile on my face.

The main indication that something strange is happening to my patients relates to the "loss of the notion of time and of space" that many of them experience during the sessions. Of these two perceptions, the loss of the notion of time is greater than the loss of the notion of space, and they assure me, for example, that they have the sensation of having been in a deep sleep for various hours when in reality only a few minutes have gone by, equivalent to the duration of my therapy. Some of them seem astonished, but not fearful about this diminution or seeming total loss of the notion of time.

Patients also often feel a sensation of pins and needles in their skin, or the presence of something strange near them; but in general they all confess that they lack the breadth of thought or the right words to describe these dimensions that are different from the purely physical and chemical sensations coming from the material world.

BIO-THERMIC VIBRATION FREQUENCIES—PATTERNS YET TO BE ESTABLISHED

The scientific proofs that confirm my therapy's ability to introduce variations in brain temperature can be seen with the analysis of the work on this subject that we did in the Colombian Air Force with that military institution's thermographic camera. These tests allowed us to observe, for example, that temperature alterations occurred in the areas my hands had passed over, at a distance of between one and two inches, without ever touching the patient.

We were even able to note that in many cases, the temperature changes were abrupt and continued after the session was over, producing variations lasting between one and three minutes, during which time the thermographic camera also registered changes in skin temperature in places my hands had approached.

What is the meaning of these temperature variations as regards the relationship that can be established to heat sources different to that produced by the effect of my therapies? The answer allows us to establish comparisons with what happens, for example, when heat is applied directly with an iron or other heating element to a body or part of a body, such as the brain. In such cases it is possible to observe a heat increase that is constant with the heat from the thermic source, and directly proportional to the increase or decrease of temperature emanating from that source, whether this be an iron, a hair dryer and/or any other electrical appliance.

With my therapy we might assume that while my hands are close to the patient the temperature likewise shows a constant increase. This, however, is not always the case, as very often the skin temperature changes of its own accord before I remove my hands, even sometimes showing phases of relative hypothermia—at others isothermal (decreasing body temperature).

This means that with my treatment we are faced with a thermic register that is not as we could have expected, in other words a temperaturebehaviour which also varies according to each patient. In addition we need to clarify that, in the majority of cases, the beginning of therapy shows an increase in skin temperature during that phase ranging between 33°C and 34°C.

What can explain this unusual temperature response on the part of the patient? The most probable hypothesis suggests a physical phenomenon: the effect of my therapy on intracranial temperature tends to increase because the intracranial cavity of the human organism contains a large quantity of liquid. When my frequencies stimulate the brain this makes it heat up, sometimes suddenly, giving rise to a process similar to that revealed in a profile of sunstroke, which as we know, generates an increase in peripheral temperature which in turn induces an internal thermic change that gives the patient the sensation of shivering.

In the case of my therapy, what is truly surprising is that, even though the patient initially registers an increase in heat, the situation can be maintained or can revert, i.e. the temperature can then increase or decrease, despite the fact that my hands continue to pass some centimeters above the patient's brain or other affected organ.

As regards the brain, sudden variations and changes of temperature and energy were recorded in each patient, which revealed a clear difference from the constant variation produced in all the patients when a heat source was involved other than that emanating from my therapy. To conclude, those changes are demonstrable manifestations that organs subjected to these therapies receive the stimulationthey need so that their cell metabolism can probably activate on its own account.

Chemistry also offers clues to confirm the validity of my therapy. In order the better to explain this I need to refer to studies undertaken a few years ago by Dr. William Tiller at Stanford University, California. His research showed that "entropy"—the greatest possible disorganization of an organism—tends naturally towards the reduction of these levels of disorganization or decomposition in the organism. Of all the models that may help us find a scientific explanation of my therapy, Dr. Tiller's is possibly the one that gets closest and is most convincing to me, and is in fact for me the one that best suits the process I deal with, which means that my frequencies would "be able spontaneously to change a state of chaos back to a state of order", in other words, to an organized state where I aim precisely to achieve this maximum result: "the regeneration and repair of the cells", and to achieve this, among other aims, in a relatively short period of time.

Nature itself is an example of the existence of negative

entropy—meaning "possessing a certain level of order"—of an auto-regulatory discipline that can be demonstrated from what has been an evolved behaviour. And this is what I refer to with my therapy: to the possibility of transferring to individuals, via frequencies, enough energies for their organisms to codify them and adapt them to their own nature, thus giving rise to "auto-regenerative responses" that allow for metabolic changes on a chemical level which are those that ultimately cure the patients.

IN SEARCH OF MORE PROOFS: THE URGENT NEED FOR EQUIPMENT AND TECHNOLOGY

The search for and discovery of more proofs to allow me to establish curing modulations in patients who undergo healing therapies refer me to the support I have received from Dr. Jorge Reynolds Pombo, pioneer in Colombia of the internal artificial pacemaker and one of the principal authorities in the world on research on the workings of the hearts of hump-back wales, on which basis his work has been fundamental for human cardiological studies.

Together with the Colombian cardiologist Augusto Leyva Samper, Dr. Reynolds has shown interest in the investigations into the therapeutic management of vibration frequencies. As such, his support for the project has been fundamental, particularly during the experiments carried out with volunteers who agreed to have frequencies applied to them while the results were recorded with infra-fed cameras in the laboratories of the Colombian Air Force (FAC). These experiments encourage me to continue investigating everything to do not only with the curative faculties of these frequencies but also, and more importantly, with the very nature and origin of these frequencies, so that we may one day copy them in order to put them at the service of medicine.

The support of Drs. Reynolds and Leyva encourages me to continue studying and analyzing with them this energy phenomenon, for which we hope to find new and more advanced equipment for interpreting the frequencies, their properties and their origins. We have reason to believe that the project demands more interest from the scientific community, if in reality we want to reach a point of no return in an investigation that should throw light on the application of frequencies which, as I have maintained all along, offer huge future benefits to humanity.

CHAPTER 4

DISEASES AND MY METHOD

EMBRIOLOGY, DISEASES AND MY METHOD—THE FETAL STATE

In previous chapters I have discussed the most accepted definition of the term healing. I have also explained the method with which I usually practice my therapy, and pointed out that healing, though not a privilege reserved to a fortunate few, requires a minimum of collaboration from the patient so that the treatment can be efficient. In the light of what has been discussed so far it is natural that we should ask ourselves how my method performs as regards the different types of disease.

According to embryology, the branch of biology that studies the embryonic development of living beings, and according to the basic classification of diseases, which divides them into ectodermic, mesodermic and endodermic types, the administration of a therapy varies from one to the other depending always on two factors: the "age" of the patients and the "time" during which the disease has been present in their organism.

Ectoderm refers to all that relates to the brain and the skin, always depending on the biological development of the human embryo in fetal state. Endoderm, from an embryological and biological point of view, refers to everything to do with gastro-intestinal and vascular disorders, while mesoderm alludes to muscular conditions, including those of the heart muscle.

The classification of diseases and the description of the method used for each disease leads us to look first at the ectoderm, that is, at the brain and the skin, these being two organs that cannot be separated from and embryological point of view.

Thus, for example, when dealing with a certain type of severe atopic dermatitis, vibration frequencies, applied in most cases to the brain, particularly when dealing with children, reveal evident peripheral changes, i.e. changes in the patient's skin.

This means that if I apply frequencies to the head of a three-year-old child with disease affecting large areas of skin, we can observe that the patient, when treatment at most has involved the thorax, experiences considerable changes and substantial improvements in other areas of the body that were not reached by my hands, such as the feet.

This all leads us to deduce that the brain is the primordial receptor *par excellence*, and that it is able to provoke positive reactions in the epithelial structure once it has received frequencies. In this case, the symbiosis between brain and skin is total.

To broaden this explanation, it is important, when dealing with neurological damage at the level of the brain, to differentiate between genetic and congenital diseases and those associated or provoked by perinatal damage. The latter are caused by damage inflicted by problems during childbirth, as for example the presence of meconium in the amniotic fluid which often leads to the so-called "fetal suffering syndrome". The list of these neurological brain damages also includes traumas and accidents.

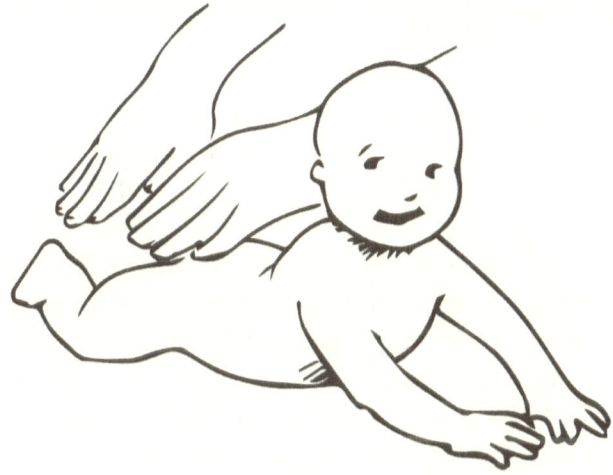

As regards the genetic origin of brain damage, the list of diseases is dominated by Down's Syndrome, where my treatment has been able to induce positive changes and substantial improvements with the respiratory difficulties often experienced by those who suffer from this disease. Equally significant changes have manifested in the cognitive development of children with this syndrome.

NEUROLOGY AND MY METHOD

In the case of congenital diseases, i.e. those associated with brain damage caused during the first weeks of embryonic time, results have been equally encouraging, because the therapy has managed to achieve satisfactory advances in cognitive and motor abilities.

In the case of diseases produced in perinatal events, specifically damage that may involve so-called "fetal suffering syndrome" during childbirth, the results of the therapy may be even more surprising as regards therapeutic procedures that are relatively easier, and this is equally true of cerebral traumas derived from certain kinds of accidents so long as the treatment is started as soon as possible.

The therapy has also shown excellent results in cases of cerebral desaturation, which is caused by a deficit of oxygen supply to the lungs due to perinatal difficulties (meconium, umbilical cord, etc.), as also with adolescents suffering from unknown types of convulsion, including epilepsy, and it has in many cases made it possible to suspend completely the use of anti-convulsive drugs.

Positive responses have also been achieved with frequency therapies in the area of certain cerebral diseases, for example transitory cerebral ischemia, all of which tend to lead to severe consequences in other parts of the body such as facial paralysis with evident complications in aphasia, dysphasia or loss or reduction of movement in arms or legs.

The best results were obtained precisely with cases of cerebral ischemia, a disease caused, as we know, by lack of oxygenation of the blood in a small peripheral artery in the brain. This tends to be transient of intermittent, which in any case means that it is a disease we could consider transitory so long as it is treated appropriately.

Cerebral ischemia can be caused by high blood viscosity or by a sudden or severe loss of blood pressure, which of course stops blood reaching the smaller arteries with sufficient pressure.

The method of conventional medicine for treating ischemia is for the artery that is transitorily closed to be re-canalized, which leads to a full recovery since in no case is this a Cerebral Vascular Accident (CVA), which always involves intracranial bleeding due to the rupture of a blood vessel (apoplexy).

Unfortunately, doctors often confuse these two conditions and give to a patient with low blood pressure a drug to lower the blood pressure even more, so that the medication practically induces a transitory ischemia. So what is important in these cases is to measure the patient's vascular circulation—hemodynamics—in order to compare it subsequently to values such as age and the presence or absence of antecedents.

If the case is of a patient over sixty years of age, the walls of the blood vessels probably present a certain degree of sclerotization, which means that there is little tonus or mobility of the vessels, so it is not advisable to lower arterial pressure abruptly with an antihypertensive, as this procedure can provoke an unwanted reduction of the levels of oxygen in some areas of the brain.

It is therefore prudent, depending on how we deal with the patient's relative inability, due to arteriosclerosis, to have an adequate tonus, to keep pressure a bit higher to avoid the incidence of a transitory ischemia, which on the other hand is very frequent in cities at altitudes over 200 meters above sea level, and is associated to habits such as a sedentary lifestyle and the use of anti-hypertensive drugs, all of which can lead to a sudden reduction of arterial pressure, an above normal desaturation and ischemia. In any case, and all the more so in climates such as our own, it is most advisable that for people of a certain age arterial pressure be kept on average a little higher, in order to guarantee enough peripheral oxygenation of the brain.

What option can my therapy propose? I try with my treatment to dilute the blood and stimulate the affected regions with my vibration frequencies, a procedure which is far from being incompatible with the processes of rehabilitation normally extended to these patients. The additional advantage of the frequency therapy is that recuperation tends to occur over a relatively brief time span, because the areas of the brain that are treated with these frequencies are fortunately more receptive, to which we can add that the process leaves no scarring or damage to the cerebral arteries.

To conclude, I am not one of those who believe that ischemia is not initially a vascular incident but rather a consequence of a thromboembolism or deficit of oxygen for a short period due to a hemodynamic reduction at a cerebral level caused very often by low blood pressure or by overdosing or excessive use of antihypertensive drugs.

We are for sure faced with a vascular incident when, in cases such as apoplexy (ACV), the effects of this type of occurrence are much more serious owing to a rupture of the artery caused by abrupt excessive hypertension, often accompanied first by an aneurism (a pathological dilation of a segment of the artery), which often leads to situations in which the person may remain unconscious and/or in a coma which eventually leads to decerebration and brain death.

Healing therapy can also be involved in the treatment of thrombosis, a term which, as we know, refers to the presence of a clot in an artery—accompanied very often by the appearance of patches of arteriosclerosis—, though the context is more difficult, specially if there are embolisms, that is to say, the breaking off of a piece that becomes known, once it has entered the blood stream, as an clot, which gives rise to embolisms.

As we said, recuperation from cerebrovascular accidents is much more complicated, which increases in proportion to the seriousness of the situation and to its impact on the affected areas, since normally the damage produced by these accidents is greater than that caused by cerebral ischemia which, as we said, is transitory. A cerebrovascular accident can in fact put an individual into a state of coma, which has a clinical profile about which we must also point out differentiation, since there are various types of coma.

Normally we speak of four types of coma: deep, medium-deep (vigil), medium-superficial and superficial. The chances of recuperation are certainly low, while the last two allow for some probability that the patient will wake up, particularly when pupil changes are observed under light stimulus.

My therapy has also shown satisfactory results in the treatment of epilepsy, a convulsive syndrome that often appears in adolescence as a consequence of traumas suffered during childhood. In the light of the treatments of conventional medicine what I have observed with this type of pathology is that, despite regular use of medication, patients often show little change in the frequency and intensity of attacks, though they often show frequent patterns of drowsiness or other neurosensory disorders.

On the contrary, the procedures applied that are founded on vibration therapies based on the management of energy frequencies have allowed for a diminution in the severity and in the periodicity with which these convulsive events follow each other. Identical results have been observed in the management of all kinds of neuralgias, such as the trigeminal nerve neuralgia (or neuralgia of the central facial nerve), or the zoster herpes that causes the so-called "shingles disease", caused by the re-activation of a variant of the herpes virus and that manifests with the appearance of tiny painful wounds that grow in ring shapes round the abdomen and other parts of the body that coincide with the corresponding segments of the affected periphery nerves.

MANAGEMENT OF SKIN, EYES AND EARS, AMONG OTHERS

However, the results that undoubtedly invite most optimism as regards the efficiency of my therapy have been in the treatment of third degree burns, particularly with children. In these cases we have been able to observe an excellent recovery of the epithelium in this type of trauma.

As regards ophthalmological diseases we have observed, especially among children, good results in the therapeutic management of amblyopia, myopia, far-sightedness and astigmatism, as also of both bacterial and viral conjunctivitis.

My therapy has in many cases been able to replace the procedures of orthodox medicine, often based on the introduction of probes to unblock the tear ducts, a procedure that is normally traumatic and painful, and also risky because of the possibilities of infection inherent in this type of procedure.

In the case of adults, *healing* therapy proves to be very efficient when dealing with infections such as neuritis of the optic nerve and glaucoma. In other cases at an intraocular level we have seen remarkable improvements including the disappearance of incipient cataracts in patients of less than sixty-five years of age.

As regards diseases of hearing, the main success has been in the treatment of hearing loss in children of less than three years, when this illness has been associated with neurosensory problems. My frequency treatment with this illness has achieved very good results, which we have confirmed with audio-metric tests following the therapy.

Acute otitis media (inflammation of the middle ear) and mastoiditis have been treated successfully with my therapy. With regard to this it is worth remembering that conventional orthodox medicine deals with acute or chronic mastoiditis with incisions aimed at draining the affected part. In this respect I remember the case of a 38-year-old patient with a Schwannoma-type neurinoma tumor; this was removed in a surgical operation that caused him months of intense pain, vertigo and nausea, none of which could be alleviated by conventional medicine. His case increased my confidence in my therapy. I remember that 90% of his pain disappeared after the first session.

In dealing with the treatment of middle otitis, application of frequencies is complemented with gentle inhalations of chamomile which allow the Eustachian tube or pharyngotimpanic tube to resume its function of balancing the pressure between the middle ear and the pharynx. Once the Eustachian tube has been reactivated the otitis quickly disappears, reducing pain and recuperating the functionality of this tube that connects the pharynx with the eardrum.

Finally, the application of frequencies is very useful in overcoming so-called "Morbus Meniere", an illness characterized by headache, vertigo and nausea, symptoms that are accompanied by high blood pressure, particularly with third age patients. It is not known what causes it, but unfortunately it is a very common complaint. My therapy attempts to balance the levels of pO_2 and pCO_2 in the brain, which considerably reduces the migraine and increases oxygenation via the blood vessels of the brain.

THE BREATHING SYSTEM AND ITS COMPLICATIONS

As regards treatment of diseases of the superior and inferior breathing tracts, *healing* has also shown itself to be very effective. With the first of these, i.e. sinusitis and pan-sinusitis, treatment includes gentle inhalations of chamomile in addition, of course, to the frequencies, which have clear and proven additional anti-inflammatory and antiseptic effects which make it easier to avoid the use of probes and other invasive procedures such as trocars. With this type of respiratory diseases the main advantage is in recuperation time, and we have documented cases where this recuperation varies from between just a few hours and a few days. The response has always been satisfactory.

As regards the other diseases of the breathing tract, the therapy is used with considerable success to treat laryngitis, pharyngitis and tonsillitis. These are infections which in the main are caused by a patient's immunological problems and we treat them with chamomile inhalations accompanied by my method, which achieve a significant and sufficiently active anti-inflammatory effect with astonishingly quick rates of recuperation.

When dealing with the inferior breathing tract (trachea, lungs and bronchial trees) I again use gentle inhalations of chamomile accompanied by my therapy. In the case of bronchopneumonia or pleurisy, the method is intensified locally or regionally, always depending on the severity of the disease.

The method has in any case had excellent results with pleurisy, bronchitis, bronchopneumonia and atelectasis, which are acute conditions which can be complemented with the application of broad-spectrum antibiotics, which would only be advisable in the case of acute bronchopneumonia diagnosed accurately and previously managed with anti-biograms and/or cultures, where necessary. It is worth noting that most diagnosed acute bronchopneumonia is viral, so conventional treatment with antibiotics is fruitless. And it is in this context that my therapy can have a positive role in overcoming this type of pathologies.

There are also very encouraging results in the case of chronic lung diseases, including chronic obstructive pulmonary emphysema and asthma, as also of certain degenerative lung diseases (such as work related diseases, including asbestosis, produced by contamination from inhalation of micro-particles of asbestos, and silicosis). We can also include lung cancer in this last category of progressive degenerative diseases. In all of these cases, my therapy has achieved improvement, though relative to how advanced the disease is.

We should not forget that in most cases, the patients we dealt with came to consultation when they were already dependent on oxygen, so that what we had to do was to improve their quality of life.

THE DIGESTIVE SYSTEM AND ITS ALTERATIONS

As regards the diseases of the stomach, and as long as the condition is not very advanced, treatment of esophagitis can be managed quite easily, as also gastric reflux, a disease caused, as is known, by a relative weakness of the cardia, the valve connecting the stomach to the esophagus that allows food through.

More difficult is treatment of achalasia, the dilation of the esophagus where it takes the shape of a funnel, which makes the patient complain repeatedly of reflux, a disease that conventional medicine confronts, when the situation becomes unsustainable for the patient, with reconstructive surgery of the esophagus. Reflux also produces worrying profiles of malnutrition.

My therapy becomes very useful in these cases, as also in the management, control and overcoming of permanent reflux in newborn children, a problem that occurs due to the weakness of the walls of the esophagus. The response is satisfactory in both cases precisely because of the insufficiency of the cardia due to the immaturity of the nervous system of the newborn child. Stimulation of the cardia with vibration energies has up till now given very encouraging results.

As with the previous case, the incidence of improvement with patients with different gastrointestinal pathologies, such as gastric erosions and ulcers that are not carcinogenic or of carcinogenic origin, has been surprising. We should mention in particular the improvement shown by patients with gastric duodenal ulcers.

In addition, I have seen major improvements in hepatic disorders, allowing for the recuperation of patients with excessive increase of transaminases, key enzymes for the organism that are produced by the liver. The results have also been very good with treatment of cirrhosis in an incipient phase, and in liver problems in general.

There are very good possibilities that the frequency therapy may become the ally of patients whose liver is seriously damaged and who are facing an imminent transplant. This reminds me of a thirty-three-year-old patient who had been offered a liver transplant as sole option, and who surprisingly managed to normalize her hepatic enzymes thanks to the frequency treatment, which allowed the transplant to be delayed for a number of months. Her case was not the only one: the great majority of persons with inflammatory of degenerative liver conditions who have been treated with my therapy have shown a decrease of transaminases which have brought these to almost or completely normal levels.

As far as gallstones are concerned, I am convinced that it is not appropriate to remove the gallbladder unless the patient is in pain.

I believe that indiscriminate surgical removal of this organ is unnecessary and indeed in certain cases it leads to permanent complicating inflammation and infections, which all affect the areas close to the gallbladder.

I should reiterate that one of the aims of frequency therapy is to make any surgical intervention be the last option in the treatment of diseases, rather than what happens nowadays, where it is the first choice of health system doctors.

As regards pancreatic diseases the panorama is undoubtedly much more complicated, particularly when we are faced with a cancer located at the head of the pancreas, one of the most lethal diseases and likewise one of the most difficult to treat. As is natural, better results are obtained from treating acute or chronic pancreatitis or type B diabetes.

DIABETES

We now make a change of scene. Diabetes, considered as the great ailment of the twenty-first century, is today one of the diseases that best reveal the harm that can be inflicted on the human organism by the noxious habits that go with modern life, such as a sedentary lifestyle and the excessive consumption of fats and sugars, which produce common charts of obesity and excessive weight in the population.

Type B diabetes can affect anyone at any moment of their life. Despite this, the results of my therapy have reduced by 80% the blood sugar levels of patients who have tested with weekly hypoglycemia curves before and after the therapies. In synthesis, I have achieved very good and quick results—from four to six weeks—when dealing with these diseases.

This being the case, and as we have seen, vibration frequencies cause rapid changes in the organism, giving rise to an increase in metabolic activity and of cell mitosis, which explains this mechanism's ability to induce cell repair and regeneration. As regards type B diabetes, I believe the therapy succeeds in achieving the required balance between the supply and demand for glucose so that the minute quantities of insulin needed by the human organism can be produced.

The successful results of the therapy are linked to brain/pancreas synchronization obtained when the glands—brain cells—receive a minimum daily dose of glucose which guarantees the improvement of diabetic patients' central metabolism and optimizing their peripheral performance. This treatment appears to contradict the dietary recommendations of conventional medicine that emphasize that all sugars be virtually eliminated.

As regards liver diseases, in addition to the successful treatment of incipient cirrhosis, we have also observed excellent results with those types of cirrhosis whose collateral effects include hemorrhaging of the esophagus, the appearance of varicose veins and the increase of enzymes called transaminase which, as we have seen, are common to many liver pathologies.

To resume, and as regards the gallstones we have already dealt with, I believe that if these gallstones do not produce complications such as inflammation of the duct of the coledochus, it is most advisable to avoid surgery in order to avoid irreversible problems.

As regards the spleen, which is responsible for the passage of blood cells, and particularly of the red globules which in part it produces, we sometimes are faced with an increase in the size of a spleen, and this is evidence of a combination of diseases of the lymphatic system, including different types of leukemia.

As we know, orthodox medicine in these cases chooses to remove the organ. In my therapy, on the contrary, I have very often achieved a normalization of the size of the spleen even when the patient has had large scale problems of the lymphatic system and even in the presence of leukemia.

As regards the intestine, subdivided into small intestine, large intestine, colon and rectum, problems can be very complex. The most common of these are connected to diverticulosis and/or diverticulitis, as well as the familiar "irritable bowel". These are pathologies which mainly appear in relatively young patients, but treatment efficiency becomes more difficult with age.

With my method I seek to obtain that the vegetative nervous system should manage synchronized peristalsis, in order to achieve a good level of reabsorption of food and an adequate hardening of the stools, so that patients are able to evacuate their bowels once or twice a day.

Of course, this type of treatments need to be complemented by the prescription of an appropriate diet, and all of this should lead to a good outcome which, depending on the time the disease has been present, could require between fourteen and sixteen weeks of sessions.

We should not forget that most of the problems we have at intestinal level are associated with the central nervous system. Thus insofar as the impulses of the nervous system are synchronized when they reach the periphery, which in this case is the intestine, we will achieve excellent results which will eliminate the most common complaints of these diseases, such as constipation and flatulence, which are symptoms of intolerance to a broad range of foods. In conclusion, what is needed is for the patient to be allowed once more to consume the foods that have been excluded by the diets they were prescribed, such as milk products and grains: chick peas, beans and lentils.

THE CORRECT USE OF NATURAL ANTI-OXIDANTS

In any case, for it to be sustainable in time, the therapy needs to be complemented with the nutritional habits recommended by the American College of Cardiology/American Heart Association. For several decades now, this has highlighted the importance of the first meal of the day being composed of a combination of fruits which, according to serious studies, are one of the best anti-oxidants, which means, among other benefits, that they diminish the toxicity of substances that we ingest every day, since they are normally present in other foods. The combination of fruits has the favourable effect of balancing the cholesterol and triglycerides that lead to arteriosclerotic type diseases.

This mixture of fruits also has the ability to convert glucose into fructose, which helps prevent diseases such as hypoglycemia, which is thought to lead to diabetes. The mealtimes recommended by the American College of Cardiology are not capricious. Research into the subject has shown that the fruit we eat during the day, that is, at times other than breakfast time, have neither the same nutritional value nor the desired anti-oxidant effects that they have during the first meal of the day.

What is more, the fibre in the fruit assists reabsorption of toxic substances and facilitates one or more evacuations during the day, guaranteeing elimination of the toxic substances and thus contributing to the cleansing of the intestines and in this manner preventing diverticulosis.

Finally, we should not forget that a bad evacuation can convert the person who suffers it into someone highly predisposed to suffering from cancer of the colon or of the rectum—or both—, which becomes colon-rectal cancer.

How, then, does my therapy function to achieve an adequate synchronicity between the activities specific to the digestive apparatus and the impulses of the central nervous system? The frequencies manage to normalize these nervous impulses, making them mutually compatible. In addition it is important to know that the disease in each organ is closely linked to the patient's age and to the time during which each ailment has been present in the organism that is being treated.

In this order of ideas, an irritable bowel affected over a twenty-year period is not the same as one that has been affected for only a few months; a similar difference exists between someone who experiences one or other disease at eighty years of age, let's say a prostatitis, as compared to someone twenty years of age affected by the same condition.

THE PROSTATE AND ITS PROBLEMS

In the case of the prostate, most patients come to my therapy with prostatism or swelling of the prostate, which frequently obstructs the urethra and causes bothersome symptoms such as the sensation of incomplete evacuation of urine, dripping after urination, weak stream when urinating, frequent need to urinate and even burning sensation during urination.

With this pathology, frequency therapy has shown that it is able to cause rapid dis-inflammation of the prostate gland, thus considerably improving urination and reducing levels of incontinence. My technique has been efficient even with patients who had previously been subjected to trans-urethral cauterizing with invasive procedures.

The success of the therapy was demonstrated by the recovery of a sixty-two-year-old patient who came to my consulting room some years ago with blood test results that revealed a prostatic antigen of 11, where the normal level at that age should vary between 3 and 4. As we know, a high antigen provides good grounds for suspecting the presence of prostate cancer, though confirmation of this requires further checks such as rectal examination and biopsy, among other aids that may indicate the presence of the disease. My patient and the patient's family were worried even further when the results of two biopsies pointed in the same direction. After six weeks of my treatment, the prostatic antigen reacted favourably to the therapy, which avoided the need for surgery that had been recommended by the doctors who initially attended the patient, a surgical process whose collateral effects often involve the persistence or worsening of urinary incontinence or erectile dysfunction, which is always traumatic for the sufferer. In any case we should not forget that, in most cases, the pharmacological treatments of conventional medicine do not work.

URINARY INCONTINENCE AND ITS POSSIBILITIES

In women, urinary incontinence tends to be a collateral effect of hysterectomy or removal of the uterus, a surgical procedure that deprives the urethra of the uterine wall on which that organ, responsible for retaining urine, rests in order to contain the urine. When the uterus is removed, the urethra loses the support it rests against, which reduces the urethral angle and therefore produces urinary incontinence.

My emphatic recommendation always tends towards the administration of non-surgical treatments wherever possible, avoiding operations that unfortunately are ordered and carried out by health systems in a way that is almost indiscriminate where there is a minimum presence of hemorrhaging to warn us of the possible presence of tumors, which are not always malignant.

THE WOMB AND IT'S QUESTIONINGS

What, then, is the advice that in my opinion should be followed by women faced with imminent hysterectomies? My opinion is that this intervention should only be undertaken where permanent hemorrhaging is causing severe anemia, the appearance of myomas and other alterations of the endometrium which over a period show themselves to be potentially dangerous to the health of the patient, which also means that other procedures, such as pharmacological medication, have failed.

My acceptance of hysterectomy is valid also for cancer of the uterus. However, in other cases such as bleeding—as long as they are treated with one or other method or therapy—, and big myomas— i.e. benign tumors in the wall of the uterus—, I recommend that hysterectomy should be avoided. Indeed, an efficient and less traumatic way to combat this type of uterine fibroid, which in all cases requires adequate annual cytology, is to await the arrival of the menopause, when the estrogen levels fall, and this in most cases allows for a normalization of the blood conditions of the endometrium.

However, this does not mean that all myomas have to disappear with the arrival of the climateric. Some will, others will not. In any case, the myomas themselves pose no threat when the patients have reached menopause and their estrogen levels have gone down.

To put this in another way, with hysterectomy the angle of the urethra suddenly changes, which means that the patient is no longer able to contain her urine. For this reason I would not advise indiscriminate recourse to this operation, nor when incontinence is the result of multiple childbirths.

With my therapy I have also had excellent results in the treatment of cystitis in third and fourth age women. This is an ailment caused by the normal appearance of rugged formations on the walls of the bladder which make a complete evacuation of urine impossible, and urination is very frequent and often painful. With this disease, urine deposits in these cavities and is held there in such a way as to cause infections which lead to the pains mentioned above.

One appropriate way to measure the magnitude of the disease requires the evidence of urograms and urodynamic tests which allow us to quantify the flow of urine that is either expelled or retained, and these tell us precisely how much urine remains inside, which favours the appearance of bacteria that lodge in the urinary duct and cause infections and the pains that characterize cystitis.

My recommendation is also against the continuous or intermittent administration of antibiotics, with which orthodox medicine treats the disease. My frequency-based therapy has managed to improve stimuli on female sphincters, on the muscle tone of the perineum and also on the muscles of the bladder walls, which has produced a better muscle coordination of the compromised organs to the extent that it helps the bladder adequately to squeeze out and expel the urine, or to reduce its accumulation to a minimum.

This muscle synchronization is achieved by applying the frequencies with one of my hands near the patient's brain, a procedure that unleashes enough stimulation of the muscle tone of the bladder, while with the other hand I manage the bactericide and antiseptic effect on the micro-organisms that cause infection. In this way it is possible to obtain total release from pain and discomfort. To obtain these results we need an average of five to seven therapies over a period of two months.

As regards ovarian diseases, we find that one of the most frequent of these, endometriosis—the appearance and growth of endometrial tissue outside of the uterus, particularly in the pelvic cavity, in the ovaries and in other parts such as the uterine ligaments or in the urinary bladder—is unfortunately poorly treated by gynecologists.

Endometriosis tends to cause considerable discomfort to those who suffer from it. Normally it is characterized by abundant hemorrhaging of chocolate coloured clots and strong colics. It produces infertility and is treated in the worst possible way by faculty medicine, whose specialists always opt for slow mutilation of the woman's urogenital apparatus, often via multiple surgical interventions and removals of the above mentioned foci of infection.

In addition, that treatment includes the use of drugs to stop ovarian production of hormones and in this way to inhibit the woman's menstruation. The effect of this type of pharmacological treatment is quite terrible, since over time it leads to severe and irreversible atrophy of the ovaries, thus adding the problem of infertility in the case of women who are young.

For this reason it is clear that orthodox medicine's treatment of this disease is excessively palliative and does not, as a result, lead to an improvement or cure. On the contrary, it leads to an ostensible loss of quality of life since it affects the woman's reproductive functions.

As a result, since this is an ailment that normally begins early on in life and gets worse with time, the recourse to extreme measures—surgical interventions and pharmacological processes—causes unnecessary ovarian damage. These conventional processes and their unwanted consequences can be substituted by and avoided with my therapy.

The explanation for this therapeutic effect can probably be traced to the origin of the disease itself, which I situate in a hormonal disorder, because the more the therapy advances the more the colic is reduced or even disappears, while the staining becomes normalized, passing from the characteristic chocolate colour to a much more normal colour. In addition, the menstrual cycle becomes normal and ovarian cysts diminish or are eliminated, with the result that in many cases there is sufficient ovulation for the woman to recuperate her fertility in normal conditions.

The presence of polycystic ovaries is usually caused by hormonal changes, a pathology that is very common in young women, unlike a malignant tumor in the ovarywhich in every case requires an exhaustive and drastic study in order to determine what procedure needs to be followed, whether surgery or chemotherapy or both. It is worth remembering that in most cases, a malignant tumor in the ovaries is extremely deceptive and therefore difficult to diagnose, precisely because it tends to be hidden, which means that therapeutic treatment almost always begins late.

The situation with benign solid cysts is different; they should be removed because they tend to grow. However, my treatment aims to manage the cyst after the malignancy has been removed, so that the main thing is to inhibit growth. The most important thing is to focus on the size of the cyst with permanent ultrasound controls and the revision of the patient's condition, because whether the tumor is malignant or benign, its growth almost always implies complications for the patient's general health.

Of course, as with many of my therapeutic treatments, how I

deal with the case depends on the age of the patient. For example, to inhibit the growth of a tumor in the case of third age women is a much safer alternative than subjecting them to surgical procedures because of the risks involved in anesthesia when a doctor has chosen this option.

If the cyst does not grow, as may be the case with a seventy-five-year-old woman, and which almost always indicates that the tumor does not have malign causes, I am able to manage the system on the basis of permanent observation with no need to rely on drastic surgical procedures. However, the surgical option is much more valid in the case of a young woman because what we prioritize in this case is that her reproductive capacity should not be affected by the presence of the tumor.

VARICOSE VEINS AND HEMORRHOIDS

With hemorrhoids, an ailment characterized by the formation of varicose veins or inflammation in the veins of the rectum and the anus, we also have to look at its most remote cause, which is related to complications specific to a dysfunction in veined reflux, which also helps to explain ailments of a similar type in other parts of the body including varicose veins in the legs.

This being the case, hemorrhoids are veins situated in the rectum wall or in the area of the anus, and they become more pronounced and also bleed with any irritation. My therapy seeks to give back to patients the stability they need for the offer and demand of blood flow, which means to adequately balance and synchronize the arterial flow with the reflux from the veins. The procedure aims to stop veins from having the greater difficulty implied in returning the veins' flow to the heart.

I achieve all this with a variety of procedures with which I believe it is possible to ensure that the heart has an appropriate control of the offer and demand of blood, with which arterial pressure is also normalized because the veins have less trouble conducting venous blood. Dealing with the problem of hemorrhoids also requires prescription of a diet and the right nutrition to avoid constipation.

Similar care is needed in treating the peripheral veins in legs and calves known commonly as varicose veins, which can be superficial or deep. This is an ailment that is dealt with by conventional medicine with surgery, which in my opinion is an antiquated method because it involves large scale removal—concretely of the safenamagna vein—which gives the patient constant cramp sensations and even more pain than that experienced before the operation.

Cauterization and extirpation of affected veins entail high risk collateral consequences. I refer, for example, to the case of a patient who before undergoing my therapy had been subjected to anal-rectal surgery to remove hemorrhoids, which left him in such a bad condition that he could not even sit down. With my treatment his case became more than satisfactory; with a single session of therapy he achieved an improvement of over 90%.

My therapy in this situation consists in activating the passive valves of the veins in order to normalize the flow in the veins and blood circulation which, in the case of varicose veins in the legs, avoids the need for orthopedic stockings. Of course, the treatment requires the patient to do a few minutesdaily exercise—such as cycling—which contributes decisively to overcoming the problem.

I use my vibration therapy in a similar fashion to deal successfully with peripheral vein ulcers, which are normally the result of a lack of vein. These ulcers tend to appear in the heel, on the inside and the outside, and are the result of problems of circulation which affect the adequate blood reflux in the tissues.

How does my therapy treat these ulcers? Normally one can observe a re-epithalization of the skin, which of course varies according to the size of the ulcer. The regenerative effects on the affected tissues and skin depend entirely on the size of the tumor and on the time the patient has had the condition.

Again, my treatment consists in bringing my hands close to the brain and also to the affected part, so that I avoid the topical procedures of orthodox medicine, such as bandages and disinfectant ointments.

Removing bandages and ointments from the affected areas also has another aim: to oxygenate the ulcer as much as possible, which makes it fundamental for the therapy to be carried out with air circulating over the area of the ulcer, which must then continue after the session is over.

We should add to the above the importance that the patient keep the affected extremity as quiet as possible. If all these conditions are maintained one can observe an improvement in a relatively short time. One or two weekly sessions lead to an improvement in almost all the ulcerous events I treat with my therapy.

I refer now to the most common diseases of the male urinogenital apparatus, I often have patients who suffer from orchitis or testicular inflammation, an ailment most commonly caused by mumps, in adult men, or also as a consequence of prostate infections or by the incidence of epidermitis. Of course this is a disease associated with sexually transmitted infections and with contagion from the ducts that are connected to the male urinogenital apparatus.

In both cases, the results of my therapy are normally very encouraging, since we have quickly managed to stem bleeding and reduce pain and inflammation in the affected testicle, which are key factors in avoiding its damage and infertility, both of which are the main consequences of this disease

These procedures are clearly different from those used by orthodox medicine which treats these episodes with antibiotics and anti-inflammatory drugs. In my case, I do away with both these solutions, and always achieve excellent results. In order to go a little deeper into this we need to remember another of the origins of this inflammation: the presence of parotitis or inflammation of the parotid glands in male adults.

BONE SYSTEM AND RELATED CONCERNS

My therapy has had good results in treating diseases of the bone system, as in the case of newborn children: hip dysplasia and dislocations in children from in very early ages (zero to twenty-four months).

Hip dysplasia, also known as "congenital hip dislocation" and today as "evolutional or developmental hip dysplasia", is defined as an abnormal development of the joint located between the thigh bone or femur and the hip, which displaces the femur outwards. In such case, that is to say, when this tendency makes the bone come out, the condition produces lameness and should be treated as a dislocation.

Hip dysplasia occurs before, during or shortly after birth in about three out of a hundred newborn babies, being most common in girls to the rate of eight out of ten cases.

My therapy treats this condition with five minute sessions once a month for at least five or six months. The therapy achieves the necessary increase in the baby's muscle tone to ensure better and more fluid internal and external rotation.

With this I aim to give the baby adequate movement of the femur towards the hip, so that it is possible to achieve a healthy bone growth of this part of the skeleton which in turn will guarantee a better and greater adaptation of the opposing bones.

In these cases my therapy achieves a better fit between femur and hip, whereby it is perfectly possible to do without the splints, plasters or surgical procedures that are suggested by orthodox medicine. As we know, common or garden orthopedics very often opt for these types of reconstructive surgery, many of which, in my experience, almost always have very limited results.

Arthritis and poly-arthritis are in this same area of ailments of the bone system, and they tend to appear in young people as a consequence of lupus erythematosus, a disease characterized by inflammation and tissue damage resulting from an abnormal performance of the immune system in which this attacks rather than protects the individual, which make it one of the so-called "systemic autoimmune" diseases.

Indeed, considering that lupus erythematosus gives its sufferers serious issues in the form of exaggerated inflammation in multiple joints and many pains, my therapeutic treatment has also achieved encouraging results, as also with other serious pathology outlines derived from the presence of this type of lupus.

I am referring to those affecting intestinal and renal functions, regarding which orthodox medicine generally relies on the administration of a broad range of cortisone and other types of immunosuppressants and steroids whose collateral effects include the possible appearance of diabetes, obesity and osteoporosis.

The great majority of my patients, especially among the young, respond very well by the end of my therapies, which greatly enhance their quality of life. The results can be appreciated after two to two and a half months of treatment.

My treatments have made it possible to reduce the doses of cortisone and the medication—including immunosuppressants in general—so that the patients experience a considerable improvement in many aspects, including when some immunosuppressants are discontinued. We should not forget that conventional treatment of the symptoms of lupus erythematosus is of an immunosuppressant type, including among others metrotexate which, in my opinion, is not advisable since it causes irreversible damage to bone marrow.

In dealing with rheumatoid arthritis, which is very frequent in individuals over forty years of age, orthodox medicine combats the disease with excessively powerful drugs, despite which it is unable always to avoid the most common deformities caused by this degenerative condition of the articulations.

In fact, because it is a progressive degenerative disease, my therapy seeks to reduce inflammation in the joints as a way to reduce pain as much as possible and improve patients' quality of life, without which they are exposed to continued use of medications, many of which cause great harm.

In these cases, logically, we explain to patients that treatment can last months, even years, with the idea that it is in any case possible to spread out the therapies in time and reduce the use of conventional medication to a minimum.

Better results are obtained when treating fractures. In most cases recuperation is possible without surgery and always with a satisfactory result. When there are dislocations as a result of accidents, my task is to try to replace the parts of the bones in the knowledge that, if there are no other possibilities, we need to think of a surgical intervention, such as with platinum implants, to permit the recuperation of the affected parts.

My therapy in these cases is based on stimulation of the osteoblasts in order to encourage the formation of a callus in the site of the fracture so as to allow the bone to settle again, and this aim needs to be permanently monitored with regular X-rays.

Despite this, it is sometimes advisable to combine the therapy with a plaster cast to guarantee that the patient keeps the affected limb as immobile as possible until healing is complete.

This is indispensable, for example, in the case of fracture of the radius, a bone that the patient must at all costs keep in the same position for a long period of time, since either flexing or rotating muscular movements risk stopping the bones from joining together again.

A plaster cast is needed or this reason and in order to guarantee immobility, while my therapy concentrates on forming a bony callus as quickly as possible. The main advantage of *healing* is that the callus is obtained very quickly. The main thing is to avoid pressure from the muscles that surround the affected bone. This pressure may not only cause intense pain but it may make it more difficult for the bone to bond to the bone facing it.

As regards osteoarthritis, my therapy has achieved highly satisfying results. As we know, osteoarthritis is a degenerative and progressive disease of the joints at osseous level, which manifests with the appearance of sclerotic plates and diminution of the intra-articular space, i.e. the space between the facing bones.

In its extreme form, when this intra-articular space is reduced, the joints naturally rub together, which makes the patient's pain unmanageable. When the osteoarthritis is at the level of the hip, and when the pain level is unbearable, conventional medicine chooses to replace the hip or the joint. This is the surgery that is commonly carried out when the patient's mobility is impeded.

Nevertheless, not all methods attempted by orthodox medicine achieve the intended results. In such cases other therapies such as mine allow for a considerable reduction of pain and improvement of the individual's mobility and quality of life.

Of course, this improvement depends to a large extent on how far the osteoarthritis has advanced in each patient. It is worth noting that the stress level caused by the pain of this condition considerably affects these patients' quality of life, and many of them assure me that they "feel they are close to death".

I must also underline that people affected by multiple osteoarthritis in different joints arrive at my consulting room with further clinical profiles, such as vascular problems, so I assume my main priority with such patients is to restore them to a quality of life that at least allows them a bit more mobility, reduces pain levels and frees them from the insomnia induced by the disease. Finally, I try to improve people's emotional state; this for the patient and for me is the most important thing.

We should not forget that when individuals are suffering as much as they do with osteoarthritis it is indispensable to treat the emotional system, and my therapy takes a very significant step in this sense. At present it is not possible to know just what happens at the level of the brain, but what I am sure of is that people's emotional state improves very considerably, which leads to a virtuous circle which to a large extent allows the patient to improve across the board.

When dealing with osteoarthritis, the treatment based on *healing* therapies tends to give contradictory signs which, contrary to what one might think, are a symptom that the patients—most of whom are women—are responding positively.

Osteoarthritis is brought on by a decalcification of the bones which normally begins with osteopenia. This disease is characterized by a significant loss of mineral bone density which is almost always a condition leading to osteoarthritis. However, not all those diagnosed with osteopenia necessarily develop osteoarthritis.

Both diseases tend to affect women more than men due to the reduction of estrogen usually due to menopause, which in turn leads to a diminution in calcium levels.

The loss of the bone minerals means that those suffering from osteoarthritis consequently sense a loss of strength in the affected bone area, which makes the bones brittle and seriously exposed to fractures. Tests used to gage the quantity of minerals in bones include those of bone densitometry, which measure bone calcium levels.

Although hormonal changes tend to appear with the onset of menopause, the risk of osteoporosis is higher after the age of fifty-five, when estrogen loss ends up affecting bone calcium levels.

For this reason, the possibility of accidents after this age almost always include even worse consequences, so prevention is always the best response to this pathology. What is more, the most common fractures affect bones that are fundamental for patients' mobility, such as femur, hips and vertebrae.

In addition to this, osteoporosis is a disease which is asymptomatic in its first phase, in other words it doesn't cause much pain on its own. Pain nevertheless appears or increases when patients are treated with my therapy. This is a normal response to the therapy which curiously reflects an improvement. The pain is caused when the periosteum, the membrane covering the bone or periost, becomes more sensitive, particularly where there are holes—which is where recalcification begins—which leads us to deduce that this is where the membrane is blistering.

The presence of pain indicates that recalcification has begun. Of course it is a pain that begins to diminish considerably after four to seven weeks. Alongside the sessions, patients should take supplements of calcium, phosphorus, vitamin D and magnesium, among other minerals that are vital to sustained recuperation.

INFECTIONS AND INFLAMMATIONS

One very important aspect in the struggle against infections concerns the electric potential of bacteria, which is affected by the bactericidal and antiseptic effects of the frequencies applied in my therapies. We here deduce that the diminution of bacterial infections is a direct consequence of this bactericide work achieved by the frequencies on those lab tests on bacterial cultures.

Of course these antiseptic bactericide results cannot be applied in the same measure in experiments undertaken with every kind of bacteria or microorganisms, because each one of those bodies has a different shell that allows it to oppose an equally different resistance to every bactericide attempt coming from the therapy.

In these cases it is possible that an infection can continue to have available bacteria even though the immunological level may be reduced. The bactericide effect of my therapy was demonstrated in relation to bacteria placed in vitro in cultures generated years before. All this does not indicate that it would have had the same results in the fight against bacterial and microorganisms because, as I said, each of these has acquired a "panzer" or hard shell to resist any intruder or most antibiotic or antiseptic agents.

Of course, we clearly need to improve the immunological level of the patients so that they achieve a system of general and not local defenses. In fact, humans live in environments surrounded by bacteria, so if we change the immunological and metabolic environment we favour the growth of the bacteria and their spread. On the contrary, if my immunological level is adequately strengthened, microorganisms or bacteria cannot harm me even though they are alive.

My theory is that immunology is part of the genetic information of each individual, and that "it can be harmed or damaged by the application of the various vaccinations". My reservations in this regard are overwhelming, and they tell me that the genes of each individual include immunological, i.e. defensive, factors that should not be complicated by drugs or by any other substance capable of altering this information.

As regards inflammation, we should affirm that most infections cause inflammations but not the contrary. This last case is included in the so-called soft inflammations, i.e. inflammations lacking in infection, such as those caused by slight bruising or other types of accident, among others.

When I combat infections with the antiseptic and bactericide components of my frequencies one would suppose that the inflammation would tend to reduce, and this does often happen. However, if I am combating a mild infection, for example the infection resulting from a rheumatoid arthritis which does not of itself involve inflammation, my focus is to attack the inflammation by reducing the tissue edema, which considerably reduces the pain caused by this type of inflammation.

This is something which I see every day in my patients, particularly those who suffer from any type of arthritis. Similar situations can present with mild inflammation caused by traumatisms and rheumatisms.

If we are dealing with an edema and seeking to reduce inflammation, the technical term we use is "chemotaxis", an ally of my therapy. In any case, the increase in enzymatic and metabolic activity is fundamental when dealing with inflammation reduction, which I achieve in most cases much quicker than is obtained with other anti-inflammatory procedures. This is quite frequently demonstrated with some cases of chronic osteomyelitis, rheumatoid arthritis and other types of traumatism.

In order to understand the role of enzymatic and metabolic activity we need to understand the role of enzymes. These are catalysts or accelerators of chemical or bio-chemical mechanisms which have the ability to unleash changes in the organism, leading to favourable effects in the human body.

In the case of an extremity, the edema causes pressure, stiffness, pain and loss of mobility. This means that these individuals experience very drastic change in a short time when they undergo my therapy. In this way, one of the greatest advantages of my *healing* therapy when compared to antiseptic anti-inflammatory drugs is the rapidity of inflammation reduction, combined with the absence of collateral damage such as that caused to the gastric system by the cortisone components that are one of the main synthetic drugs used to treat osteomyelitis.

And as occurs with the rest of patients of other pathologies, one of the main symptoms of improvement, in addition to inflammation reduction, is the sensation of thirst, which is one of the characteristics that accompany this recuperation. Recovery of mobility is also relatively quick.

The inflammation also gives us clues, not always very precise ones, as to the presence of other diseases, sometimes serious ones such as cancer, so that even though inflammation reduction is an aim to be pursued, it is essential to try to discover what type of tumor we are dealing with, that is, if it is malign, semi-malign of benign. This is important because processes of inflammation and inflammation reduction tend to be almost identical to those that cause the infections.

TUMORS AND THEIR TREATMENT WITH MY METHOD

It is possible with my therapy to improve a patient's clinical profile even in the case of cancer, by reducing inflammation and eliminating the pain of the tumor. However, it is not always possible to change the direction of growth of the tumor, which can continue to ramify. Even then, in other cases of cancerous tumors it is possible to slow down rapid tumor growth, even to inhibit it completely, as compared to other therapeutic treatments.

As regards semi-malign and benign tumors, my therapy can not only improve the general situation by reducing inflammation and pain, but in so doing can also revert the disease, particularly in organs such as ovaries and testicles. However, semi-malign and benign tumors must not be under-estimated, for although they do not have a malign component, their growth is invasive and infiltrative, as with neurinoma, Schwannoma and meningioma. Although benign, such tumors have an internal growth that presses on the brain or other vital organs.

In the case of bone diseases, our reader needs to know first of all how modern science groups the diseases of the skeleton into three categories: 1) infections and/or inflammations; 2) degenerative diseases; and 3) diseases caused by traumatisms. As regards traumatism, that is, when we are talking about fractures and their consolidation, I need to say that *healing* therapy has proved itself effective in accelerating the ossification of the fractured parts.

This ability to recuperate rapidly is directly proportional to the type of patient who has suffered the fracture. Thus it is that newborn babies show a quicker inflammation reduction in tissues and bone ossification or consolidation.

It is of course essential with fractures to ensure, with the use of splints and plaster casts in the case of dislocation, that the affected part is immobilized. In extreme cases, osteosynthesis is acceptable when it is a case of completely repositioning the bone. Osteosynthesis is above all a surgical support that uses plates to hold affected extremities in place. It is nevertheless possible that a patient, after osteosynthesis or an implant, might develop osteomyelitis, which in other words is an infection of the bone characterized by the presence of a focus of infection, by inflammation of surrounding tissues and by acute persistent pain that does not lessen even after treatment with antibiotics and anti-inflammatory drugs.

On this score I should mention the case of a sixty-six-year-oldpatient who suffered or developed severe osteomyelitis having fractured his elbow ten years previously, with repositioning osteosynthesis by means of various wires to join the separated fragments.

Swelling of the tissues and pain brought him to my consulting room some months ago, since when he has made a remarkable recovery. *Healing* therapy allowed him to suspend antibiotics and anti-inflammatory drugs. My therapy involved approaching my hands to his head and his arm, which reduced the inflammation and infection in the area; simultaneously, small bone fragments, that had been floating in the tissues and causing pain, managed to consolidate.

Osteomyelitis is not a disease we should underestimate, as it can lead to amputations when, in the case of an extremity, it is treated incorrectly by conventional medicine.

As regards arthritic diseases, two of the most common conditions that afflict my patients are rheumatoid arthritis and lupus erythematosus, which we mentioned earlier. Rheumatoid arthritis is more common in women than in men, and tends to develop after the age of forty and leads over the years to grotesquely deformed joints that make mobility difficult. Lupus is more common in girls than in boys, and the symptoms normally appear during adolescence.

As for arthritis, the results of my therapy are very encouraging. Positive reactions to treatment can be observed after eight to ten weeks from beginning treatment, with considerable relief from pain and visibly reduced inflammation of the joint. Even then, people tend to complain a certain amount during the first two or three sessions, which paradoxically confirms to me that the treatment is proceeding as intended. 98% of my patients react favourably to the therapy, but in all cases the patient needs to understand that there may be an increase in pain in the first stage of treatment.

Results are better in the treatment of lupus, an autoimmune disease—i.e. where the immune system attacks rather than protects the patient. Of all autoimmune diseases, lupus is one of the easiest to manage with my therapy. If it is systemic, lupus affects joints and kidneys and other organs such as the colon.

As regards degenerative diseases of the bone system, one of the most frequent is osteoarthritis, an intra-articular sclerosis of the facing parts of two bones.

In addition to the surgical interventions that traditional medicine chooses to deal with this disease, sufferers choose other therapies, some of them dating back to the classical Greek period. Indeed, for centuries, people have tried to control the pain of osteoarthritis with thermal baths and the appliance of hot sulfuric mud. These palliative treatments do in fact relax the muscles, which in turn lessens pain.

There are also the Finland waters and the Kneipp's baths, the latter discovered by the German monk Sebastian Kneipp, born in Bavaria in1821, who successfully treated tuberculosis with this therapy in the nineteenth century. Kneipp's baths involve alternative applications of hot and cold water, which produce positive physiological changes which allowed this monk to overcome tuberculosis, despite the seriousness of that disease, and to maintain an improved quality of life, to such an extent that forty-five years after suffering the disease, his autopsy did indeed detect signs that he had suffered from tuberculosis.

This therapy quickly gained prestige for its successes in the nineteenth century, so that various personalities, such as Pope Leo XIII, sought Kneipp to gain the benefits of his therapy, and experienced the same recovery as its inventor.

RECOMMENDATIONS

As regards the most common children's diseases, I should mention how, at home, we can deal positively with certain cases where intense pain, and the fact that the child is unable to describe the symptoms of its distress, often make parents worry uncontrollably over the symptomatology. We should remind ourselves that if adults deal wrongly with these pains the child can be hospitalized unnecessarily, and the child's condition can be made worse precisely because of the hospitalization, generally at night, none of which assists its recuperation even though we may be reassured to see that the child is stabilized in the hands of the doctors.

We should note that I have used the term "stabilized" and not "cured", because very often what we obtain in a hospital is not a sustained improvement of the child's condition but its stabilization, after which it is very common for the symptoms or other ailments to recur. For sure, errors are common in the identification of illnesses when diagnoses are made in an emergency department, due among other factors to the anxiety of parents and doctors focusing on the symptoms rather than the illness.

Because the aim is to combat the child's pain, how to overcome the underlying illness is often not identified, so the child is very often taken repeatedly to the emergency units of our hospitals, clinics and health centers, whatever level that medical institution may have.

Otitis media: One of the clinical profiles that results in most emergency hospitalizations is otitis media, a disease characterized by sharp pains in the ears, accompanied by fever. The main recommendation for these cases is to block the ear with cotton wool and to avoid using eardrops. The most important thing is to do direct inhalations of chamomile, considered to be one of the best natural anti-inflammatory agents. If the child is a baby it is best to put the steaming pan next to the cradle so that the child can inhale the vapours without difficulty. The aim of this treatment is to reduce inflammation of the larynx in order to restore the balance of pressure between the middle ear and the pharynx through the Eustachian tube.

As regards bronchial or lung infections with coughing, expectoration and noises in the chest during breathing, accompanied by mild fever—as long as the expectoration is not of a yellow-green colour—then it is a viral infection and in most cases treatment can take place at home, but it is not prudent to use antibiotics. We recommend rather that the child be treated for several hours with chamomile inhalations—placing the stove at some distance from the child or baby's bed. This is a simple home remedy that should be repeated for three days by placing a pan with a lot of water and chamomile at low heat to increase the room temperature to an average of between nineteen and twenty-one degrees centigrade. The effect is achieved by leaving the pan on the heat source in order to hydrate the air with the steam of the water that comes off it.

If there is sputum—that is to say, when the expectorant turns green or yellow—we can deduce that there is a mixed infection. In this case, depending on its seriousness, one can consider the use of antibiotics. But from my experience, even in these events we can do without antibiotics by using chamomile, thanks to the excellent anti-inflammatory properties of this plant. In fact we now know that for the treatment of this type of disease, antibiotics have insufficient bactericide properties or ability to inhibit the growth of the colonies of bacteria. What is more, where there is high fever the child should never be bathed in cold water. I prefer the child to be cleaned with damp towels and be left wrapped up in light sheets taking care not to allow air to enter the room from outside.

Except in cases of very high fever, we can place bandages moistened with iced water on the child's forehead, temple or armpits, as long as we have checked that these are hot because of the fever. This is because the rest of the body is not necessarily affected by the fever, since temperature is not usually constant across a human organism.

On the other hand, consumption of water should increase in proportion to the behaviour of the fever as it also increases. In other words, the more the fever, the more there should be consumption of water. Food, on the other hand, should be provided as the fever goes down, with the aim of preventing the stomach from filling with heavy nutrients. Light soups and soda biscuits in the intervals of low fever are always advised in these cases. Normal food intake should only be resumed insofar as the fever is reduced to normal levels. For the patient to make a better recovery, chamomile plays a fundamental part, since it is an excellent natural anti-inflammatory agent, as we said before.

Cough: Pathological profiles associated with persistent coughing, whether dry or with expectoration, also require differentiated treatments for each case, which implies knowing precisely the symptoms of each.

We will deal first with dry coughing, known as croup. This is an extremely sudden occurrence that brings the child in a couple of hours to a state of breathlessness, which in turn, understandably, causes the parents to become frantic, often forcing them to take inappropriate measures. It is a very common disease in the high plains, where the patient's evolution can become critical so quickly that it becomes urgent to take the child to an emergency unit, where almost always tubes are inserted. However, risks of infection are not uncommon or superfluous, so we should remember that these patients can improve with home remedies that will avoid dragging the child around, making its condition worse, putting tubes in it or putting it in hospital, often with disastrous consequences since there is the danger of desaturation and later neurological problems.

The process is very simple. Various recipients with a lot of vaporizing water should be placed next to the child's bed, along with wet sheets in the room. One can use a small amount of corticosteroids (5 milligrams of prednisolona), which in less than two hours will bring about a considerable change in the child's breathing and a reduction in the dry cough, which is a metallic-sounding cough commonly known as dog's cough.

Croup, or membranous laryngotracheitis, is a severe inflammation of the larynx, which can be reversed with hydration of the child's entire environment, so that the key is to saturate the child's room with hot water.

Dry cough: should be treated with a simple inhalation of chamomile several times a day. The elimination of sputum is important for this type of ailment, so it is good to give the child an additional natural expectorant to assist with this expulsion. The infusions or vaporizations of chamomile moisten the superior and inferior respiratory tracts, thus helping with these expulsions.

Vaporizations for other types of cough, as also to combat pulmonary disease, should ideally be applied during the night or at nightfall. Vaporizations should not be applied directly in the baby's face, which is extremely irritating for the child's nostrils and also risks burning its face with the steam.

Diarrheas: Where there is a profile of diarrhea we recommend giving the patient carrot juice. This is a very effective home remedy with most of these profiles, whatever the age of the patient. The preferred method is to prepare the juice with an extractor. Otherwise one method is to boil a pound and a half of carrots until they soften, then to strain them, add sugar and eat them immediately. Most diarrheas are caused by adenovirus that bring about intestinal disturbances. Serum, of course, helps combat dehydration but is not enough to halt the diarrhea. Very light soups and carrot juice contribute to the remission of the diarrhea until the patient is fully recovered. The main thing, however, in addition to halting the diarrhea, is to make a correct diagnosis of the origin of the disease. The dosing can be suspended when the patient has recovered. When there is vomiting, anti-emetics should only be used in very severe cases.

Bleeding hemorrhoids: In these cases, it is advisable to opt quickly for a change of diet, giving the patient soft foods that produce a soft stool once or twice a day, which eliminates rigidity in the fecal matter which makes the hemorrhoid sufferer's condition worsen. The bleeding can of course be treated by washing the anus with hot water after each deposition. This washing should be done without soap, and dried with clean cotton wool. A topical ointment can then be applied, which will help avoid infections and reduce inflammation in the affected veins.

Hip dysplasia: This is an ailment that affects girls more than boys, and parents can contribute decisively to their child's recuperation. My therapy is not a procedure that needs to be applied urgently, but it has shown itself to be highly efficient in treating this ever more common problem. Daily swimming and tricycle riding help improve muscle tone and mobility in the legs (that is to say, with the bone's abduction or inward and outward rotation). This stabilizes the affected joint and in the medium term reduces the affected angles in the children's hip.

CHAPTER 5

HEALING: SOME
PHILOSOPHICAL IDEAS

ABOUT DEATH

Up till now we have noted how *healing* therapy is able to deal successfully with a broad range of diseases of different types, with the clarification that this depends on factors such as the age of the patient and the length of time that it has manifested with the individual. It is even more evident that *healing* is a therapy focused mainly on attacking the causes and not the symptoms of diseases, so my work aims fundamentally to unleash the mechanisms of the human organism itself to attack these causes. It would nevertheless be very pretentious to maintain that the *healing* therapy prioritizes the battle against disease even when this is of a definitively incurable nature.

Healing therapy is certainly not at the service of eugenics, that is to say, at the service of medical procedures of any kind that prioritize maintaining life mechanically when it has finished, which is the opposite of euthanasia, but just as immoral. What I have observed with many of my patients, and to my great satisfaction, is that when death is imminent they feel infinitely more at peace with the therapy than without it. These experiences have also been reported to me by family members of patients close to death having received my therapies during their illness.

Their witness reports that at the moment of death these patients show "a better mien", are emotionally balanced and often enter into a state of indescribable ecstasy.

My general opinion regarding thanatology, in the sense given to this term, i.e. "the study of death", is based on my many experiences with patients at varying stages leading up to death, as also on many long conversations with doctor friends who have had similar experiences.

My general impression is that human beings lack a clear sense of the inevitability of death. Effectively, our ignorance of what awaits us after life is over prevents us from approaching death more naturally. Death is something that cannot be negotiated, yet despite this, humans are so attached to life, to material things and to what they have around them, that they refuse until the last moment to admit this imperative.

Man, particularly in Western culture, never or seldom thinks that death is not just an inevitability; it is in some sense an unknown alternative. He has never taken on board that the end of life can also be a solution.

Undoubtedly it presents us with a change of reality, in the sense that we have to pass from what we know to what we do not know. Fear of this passage leads to mental disquiet that can block the organism from making a peaceful transition towards death. Let us not forget that the brain itself gives the green light to this moment. To understand this can facilitate the inevitable passage towards death, which requires a mental preparation to allow the human being to attain, as far as possible, a welcoming transition.

Personally I have known very few people who have been able in this way to relinquish life and the material world that we know. My feeling about this is that those who achieve this are somehow people with an astoundingly clear conscience of death, close to a feeling of yearning where the foremost thing is a conscious and eager search for a different level, probably superior, in which the absence of pain is in itself an incentive.

It is not just the expectation of a life after death, which is something which possibly depends on the faith of each person, but is the option death represents for someone who glimpses in pain the imperfection of human life.

These patients somehow glean a sense that the life they have lived has not given them enough to be happy, and they have the profound conviction that life will not make them happy in the same way as they hope to achieve happiness in that other dimension into which with stoicism they desire to enter.

These are patients that I would not situate in the realm of depression. They are, in fact, not depressed, and they demonstrate a certain emotion at making the transition to where they will find a happiness that they assume to be greater or different to their earthly lives. They experience a certain lethargy as regards the different situations of their life and they have embraced with some pleasure the idea of a journey about which they show themselves to be sure.

Of course, to attain this type of transition from life to death, from the known to the unknown, requires from us a deep awareness that our natural clinging to life must be so rational and limited that it must not close us to the idea that death is a step and not the end. All these reflections and experiences are probably what have allowed me to expel from my vocabulary the term "terminal patient", because I believe that this is an idiomatic expression that mistakenly emphasizes the idea that death is the end of everything, the moment when everything finishes and nothing begins, and I insist that this is repugnant to me and is an unethical factor in the doctor/patient relationship.

However, "terminal patient" is unfortunately a much used concept in orthodox medicine. I believe it is not terminal, in that I believe that the ending of cellular life does not signify the sudden ending of the scope of energies. Energy is not something that ends, but something that continues on other levels unknown to us.

"Terminal" suggests that all is finished, but I definitely believe that not to be the case.

I therefore believe that we must constantly prepare ourselves at this level, which implies shedding many of the concepts of our education. For sure, the idea of an afterlife, an "eternal life" in correct Christian parlance, has been sold to us for centuries. This has been based on faith and not on reason, so the apprehension of death as an inevitable step towards the unknown remains the preserve of spirituality.

But the fact is that not all cultures have the same attitudes towards death. There is the case of certain Hindu monks who literally choose the moment to die by means of what they call "the act of separating the soul from the body", and this seems quite strange to us.

In such cases we can talk of a kind of ecstasy, of an emotion that frees us from all harm to reach consciously and pleasurably towards death. This being the case, these people seem able to conjure up the ecstasy, that state of someone seemingly outside the world of the senses, in a trance, in the state most close to death.

Ecstasy is therefore a tool that enables all human beings to enter into another consciousness, which because it combines mind and spirit, should allow us also to enter into a trancelike state.

In any case I believe that the attainment of ecstasy is a faculty that all beings should be able to develop, but of course we need the will to attain it. Preparing for our death is not something that can be so mechanical for us. The importance of learning the art of dying means that we should prepare ourselves for it from childhood and that this perspective be continued through adolescence, so that education plays a fundamental part. When all is said and done, death is always imminent.

ABOUT REINCARNATON

Logically, there are some peoples across the world who are more involved with a philosophy and a religiosity that make them more open to accepting death. Some of them rely on reincarnation and see in death a permanent step to the life they have left.(Do you mean to a new life?)

To conclude, it is fundamentally important to educate the peoples of the Western world regarding the importance of preparing human beings for this irreversible situation of death, and educate minds pedagogically to assume this responsibility in relation to these situations, in relation to themselves and their family members, however painful that may be. I feel that today's doctors lack precisely this ability to guide the patient through this step, the last of their life. Their inability is perhaps founded on that narrow view that constantly reminds doctors that their mission is to cure disease, ignoring the fact that doctors, faced with the impossibility of curing some diseases, cannot be relieved by priests, but that both doctors and priests must commit to that holistic support that is needed by human beings when they near their end.

In synthesis, it would also be right for doctors to offer their patients this important support, even though we do not belong to societies where our sense of life is permeated with acceptance of death. Doctors should have a special sensitivity that allows them to prepare their patients for the proximity of death.

Unfortunately there are many doctors who are ill-prepared to assist their patients in this way. But the contrast with obstetricians is of significance. When a child is born, the obstetrician usually holds its hand, and this is something that very few doctors do when a patient is nearing death. We must require doctors to help dying patients in sensitive ways and that, by the same account, they abstain from torturing them when there is nothing that can humanly be done for them. Their role, in this case, should be to guide them with advice on how to accept the situation.

My therapy has on several occasions been very useful in making death easier for a patient, insofar as it has efficiently contributed to this end by eliminating pain and reducing stress and the levels of anguish, anxiety and depression that tend to affect individuals nearing death.

I have observed with satisfaction how many of these patients assume a positive and favourable attitude towards what awaits them. There have been several cases where the pleasant feelings induced by my therapy have been evident. I remember, for example, the case of a Venezuelan woman who, according to the witness given by her family members, was "able to see me in her room" shortly before her death, when in reality I was thousands of kilometers away. Such cases of bilocation are sometimes common in these situations. But what most surprised me of that case was the way she died, for she was able to say good-bye to each and every one of her family members, and then, with an expression of profound tranquility, to die peacefully without the least sign of anguish.

My therapy's ability to mitigate pain with this type of patient was confirmed to me with the death of a woman doctor in Bogotá's ClinicaCorpas. I had treated her for muscular cancer from 1997 to 1998. The sharp pains she suffered could not even be controlled with the high and increasing doses of morphine that they gave her each day. After just one of my therapies this woman needed no more morphine, and went into a state of relaxation that lasted until her death, which occurred in total tranquility a few weeks later.

It is worth insisting on why I oppose the term "terminal" that is widely used in orthodox medicine when referring to patients who are close to death. I believe, effectively, that we cannot speak of "terminal" when what I can vouch for in the organism is that at a certain point the workings of the cells and with them the physiological functions of the human body come to an end, but not what relates to energy.

The energy component is not, in fact, something that comes to an end with the end of the cell functions, but that continues at other levels unknown to us. To leave this beautiful possibility open is therefore a task that the health professional should constantly transmit to the patient. Not to do so is to accept that "terminal" means that everything comes to an end. Consequently, it seems to me to be a term that is too absolute and that leaves no room for the idea that there is "something more", and that therefore what has come is not an end.

Of course this is not a new argument, yet it is not sufficiently known and assimilated in the Western world. Buddhist philosophy, for example, tells us graphically of a wheel that goes from top to bottom: it is the continuity of the being in its most holistic dimension. "Terminal", I repeat, has an excluding meaning that allows for no alternative to the implication that the end is total.

ABOUT LIFE AFTER DEATH

I will not delve very deeply into what I believe awaits us in the afterlife precisely because I do not want to be part of that bibliographical "boom" where hundreds of books tell us each year about suppositions and supernatural experiences that are undoubtedly received with much interest by thousands of people throughout the world, quite legitimately anxious to decipher anything about what happens after death.

This is a dangerous tendency insofar as it lends itself to risky manipulations at a social level. We have only to remember the suicides that took place in the USA because of theories that irresponsibly held out the possibility of travelling with extraterrestrials, based on the astronomical phenomena that occurred at the time with comets passing through the solar system.

What is needed, then, is a serious and responsible position on these matters. I feel there is an overdose of books and films that generate false expectations about our fate after death

I suggest we focus consciously on the situation we are living in, which I feel requires that we identify the legacy and mission that we each have and find out how we can fulfill it. The satisfaction we get from fulfilling this legacy is to seek the happiness of others. We all have to reach a conclusion.

Whether or not we are fulfilling this mission is essential to our being able to take a position, as yet unknown to us, regarding death. The challenge now is to try to fulfill that mission. Only then will we be able to generate transformations at a level of awareness of death.

This being the case, and as it affects my therapy, the aim is not only to seek the happiness I can give my patients by providing improvement in the state of their health. In addition I seek to lead them to a deep reflection and to unconscious and subconscious ways of thinking so that people are able to take full charge of the value of life.

My idea, somehow, is to insert into my patients a new "chip" to deal with life and death. It is a question of broadening people's awareness that life, in some ways, is the result of what we make of it, and that a heightened awareness of the non-negotiable fact of death can give us keys for living better.

This new awareness of health and of life eventually leads my patients to acquire better tools for dealing with each day as it comes, without that death-related anguish that affects people's quality of life both in health and in sickness.

I base the evidence that this is possible on what I am told by family members of those facing death. In almost every case these deaths have been peaceful, tranquil, free of anxiousness and depression. They have expressed gratitude towards life, towards those close to them, towards me.

My own mission as I develop my therapy goes beyond that of calming pain, which is of course an ethical obligation stemming from the Hippocratic Oath. I also aim to seek the cause of sickness and to eliminate it, in order to allow the mechanisms of nature itself to act in favour of the patient's sustainable recuperation.

Together with this it is fundamental to deal rightly with emotion, to resist anguish and to provide patients with the happiness they need in order to prepare for death, even on the basis of respect for and enhancement of their beliefs when they assume that reincarnation offers hope for continuity.

In this sense, and only when patients understand that their life transcends the life of cells, will I give them tools to meet the challenges implied by a life of health and a death with dignity.

What is important, then, is to give life a higher meaning in order to approach a healing that is not only of the body but is multidimensional, a concept that no doubt leads us to accepting that there are other possibilities beyond material life.

But what are these dimensions? To answer this question I need to rethink what I myself have been throughout my personal and professional life, and this is an exercise that will not be entirely valid unless I share with my reader the story of my origins and of why, towards the end of the 1970s, I devoted myself to medicine in the bucolic scenery of the Austrian alps.

MATTER-ENERGY SYMBIOSIS

It is no simple matter to understand these dimensions of energy, in that for thousands of years we have seen both the material and the spiritual worlds as absolutes, as two areas of human existence in relation to which we refuse to include life energy manifestations capable of acting to benefit both matter and spirit.

However, to approach the world of energy vibrations and its many applications represents new challenges and a few problems. One of these relates to the existence of a dimension existing between matter and spirit, and breaks with the immutability of the "law of opposites", that sort of binary opposition that for centuries has allowed us to reduce the world to a succession of bi-polar concepts that speak of night and day, matter and spirit, life and death, black and white, and heaven and hell. This is a rigid succession that leaves little room for other options such as one that would allow us to understand the presence of dimensions of energy whose existence we cannot deny just because we are unaware of them.

But the problems don't end here. In my opinion, to be connected to vibration frequencies of this kind, whose origin as we have said is unknown, places me in a position that is difficult to explain, particularly because of the what I still experience as a dilemma, namely to know if this faculty makes me a privileged being. I still find it impossible to state precisely whether this gift makes me someone different, which on principle I reject as I am convinced that everyone can somehow establish a connection with this type of vibration. What I obviously do not know, and this I freely admit, is what conditions are required for someone to channel vibration frequencies for the purpose of therapeutic procedures.

The above refers me to insist once more on the need to look deeply at everything to do with the probable origin of these frequencies. I believe that the closest model for pinpointing the origin of these frequencies can be found in the complexity of our cosmos—I refer to the great numbers of radiations and/or frequencies, known and unknown, that are permanently reaching Earth from all over the universe. Effectively, it is about the thousands or perhaps millions of radiations and manifestations of energy that are received by large radio-telescopes round the world.

All this allows me to conclude that somehow, since we are living beings, we form part, even though on a minimal scale, of that complexity of the universe. We can deduce, specifically, that some of those radiations may be energy frequencies upon which all the precursor elements of earthly life have settled. If we observe the most recent research carried out in 2009 with powerful radio-telescopes, its conclusions throw up clear signs that within a few decades should lead to the confirmation of this theory.

But of course, if we are talking of the precursors of life on Earth, we must think that these precursors are obviously supremely appropriate frequencies that are perhaps far superior to the radiations of our solar system. There is also the possibility—I do believe—that the great number of inexplicable phenomena that have accompanied us throughout our human history may be explained on the basis of these vibration frequencies.

I am referring, for example, to paranormal phenomena such as levitation, which clearly cannot be explained as types of magnetic or electromagnetic energy yet which in any case escape our frameworks, be they physical or non-physical.

If we start from the latter possibility we can also arrive at physical equations more advanced than those of Albert Einstein who, as we know, established that the greatest speed that a human may ever reach will always be less than the speed of light. Of course, what type of physical realities can be constructed on the basis of Einstein's theories will take a very long time to establish. In the meantime what is really important is to become aware of and to strive to focus on Einstein's theories in a way less absolute than we have so far.

This will allow us to approach the idea that "energy is information", and as such it travels and is permeable to transformation. In this line of reasoning, it is possible to think that the transformation of energy is produced in an ascending fashion, so that it will be possible in the not too distant future to obtain new information, and that this will allow us to better manage our relationship with the universe.

For now, energy as information only seems close to us if we consider the realities of our daily existence in which it has been possible to put electro-magnetic waves at the service of human communication in the form of satellites and antennae that code and de-code data, texts and videos via countless gadgets that form part of our daily life, such as cell-phones, TVs, etc. This allows us to understand how, two hundred years ago or less, there would have been outright astonishment at the thought that information, images or voices could travel or be seen or read in another hemisphere thousands of kilometers from their point of origin.

Humans are the creators of this means of manipulating that information, and have developed the ability to transmit it from one place to another. On this basis, why not think of the existence of frequencies with properties greater than those known and used up till now? Personally I believe that the volume of information that can travel through these vibration frequencies is greater that all we know at the moment. It is in this realm that we can think that this information is even capable of generating in the human organism mechanisms of body auto-regulation that can cure diseases.

The search for signs of the existence of these types of cosmic frequency and their incidence in the material plane known to us poses complex problems, but also encouraging scientific expectations. For now, radio-telescopes have brought us signals of cosmic frequencies unknown at molecular level, which according to researchers could be the precursors of life on our planet.

In fact, recent experiments with the particle accelerator lead us away from the scientific bases that situate the beginning of all to the impact of solar energy in our planetary system. This suggests the idea that the solar system might not be the cause or origin of all our known biological life.

All this reflection leads me to believe that cell repair—in this case, of the human organism—is also quicker than that produced by magnets and currents produced by artificial magnetism. In short, one effect of the existence of these frequencies would be linked not only with cell repair but also with the incredible speed at which this has been documented with healing therapies.

This also brings us close to Franz Mesmer's theory we mentioned earlier, when he spoke, 200 years ago, of the existence of "a magnetic fluid of cosmic type". I agree about the cosmic element, but not about magnetism; I believe Mesmer was right in everything except the magnetic manifestation of this cosmic fluid. I believe that Mesmer, as other healers throughout history, did indeed deal with cosmic frequencies of unknown origin that had a variety of properties and information far superior to what is known to us.

It also seems to me that this could explain the symbiosis or connection that exists between multiple energies that have evolved and transformed into rich information capable of intervening in all biology as we know it. The challenge, of course, is to obtain equipment that is more sophisticated than the radio-telescopes and will some day be capable of measuring non-magnetic frequencies.

MAN, UNIVERSE AND GOD: SOME PERSPECTIVES

If we deal with themes related to healing we face a problem common to all cultures insofar as spontaneous curing and healing have so far been seen as gifts with a divine manifestation and origin. This gives us an idea of how difficult it is for a therapist to work in the area of healing. And this is a problem without a solution, because in all societies, the material world is the domain of the living being, while other domains such as the spiritual domain appear to be reserved exclusively as the world of mysticism and religion.

Because of this it is important to devote some lines to the arguments used by healing therapists such as myself to confront the issue. In earlier chapters I mentioned that the benefits of *healing* are not reserved to believers and are not the privilege of a specific religious creed.

I have also been forthright in saying that my faculty of healing does not make me an extraordinary being nor anything of the sort, since the distinction is already clear between *healing* based on this type of frequencies and experiences that are absolutely impenetrable to human understanding.

It is not easy for therapists, whoever they may be, to have to refer to a subject so personal to each of us as is faith and belief in matters supernatural. But it is important to clarify that our own idea of God is something personal, and in my case I am moved to think of the Creator as a "maximum nucleus of energy" from which all else derives. This is to venture towards careful reflections that are inevitably connected to our personal cosmovision.

What role can be reserved to God, as a maximum expression of energy, in *healing* processes based on the application of vibration energies? This question implies a problem insofar as it would seem to propose a link between this type of energy and the idea of a God who intervenes in our daily life, which would include the curing of our illnesses, as is visualized by some Pentecostal—and Catholic charismatic—movements, which see a God who intervenes in our health and sickness and in many other aspects of our daily life.

The hierarchy we give to the concepts of God, Universe and Biology—in which latter category we humans are included—contributes to solve the problem on the basis that God, as the maximum fount of energy, exists, though in relation to this we cannot deduct with precision if the power of *healing* comes directly from Him or from the frequencies of cosmic nature, which of course may some day be measured and known by human beings.

A different point of view would be that of hoping that the cosmic vibrations originate in that "Einsteinian idea" that we have of God.

With this in mind, further questions are raised. Is the universe always matter? Is the universe synonymous with visible reality or can we include in it the intangible world? If we accept the idea that the universe somehow incorporates the realm of matter, are we not getting close to the concept that God, as maximum expression of energy, is part of the universe? If this is the case, are we not perhaps on a theoretical plane in which God and the Universe are one and the same, or quite the contrary, can we not move towards the idea that the Creator is the maximum source of cosmic energy, which would lead eventually to the idea that God is the last level of a scale of energies from which all other energies flow?

This is not a philosophical treatise, so I tend to think that the physical-morphological realm is provided with a structure that somehow ties it in with the intangible, which for me is the realm of energy. So here we enter upon all that links and separates matter and energy.

According to Einstein's model, any energy can be converted into matter, in the same way that any matter can be converted into energy. This leads us to a more evolved thought, which allows us to conclude, along with many scientists, that our sun has no connection to the origin of life.

As a morphologically tangible structure, the universe probably hides a few secrets over and above those that matter has revealed to us. On the same score, why not think that on the basis of that matter there are other energies that are obviously unknown? We are, in other words, looking at a primary model that leads us to a more complex question.

We, as living beings, are also part of this universe that is matter, and this means we are provided with a morphology that is tangible, but also structured, as I said before, in such a way that we are obviously connected to the intangible, to what I call the realm of energy.

Our brain at this moment in time is matter, which traces limits to each human being and gives us all an equal ability to visualize the material world. Of course if we had a different morphological structure we could see things differently. And since questions spring up around everything, we can ask ourselves if God created us to see Him this way. If that is the case, then Darwinian biological evolution would not deny the existence of God, as happens today in the USA with the Manichaean and irreconcilable divorce between Creationism and Evolutionism. In my opinion this evolutionary scheme is based on a source of energy that is protected by a plan of creation that holds that the Supreme Being wants to see us evolve permanently so that we can see Him as we do at present.

In this sequence of ideas, I would believe that our own scientific evolution allows us to advance towards a greater knowledge of those energies wherein it is possible to perceive God as something more tangible and reasonable, as opposed to the un-reasoned idea of Him proposed by many cultures and religions throughout the history of mankind.

I personally believe that the universe has a balance between the material and the so-called immaterial worlds. We know the universe itself, albeit precariously, but I would prefer to replace the concept "immaterial" with that of "antimatter", insofar as the latter fluctuates with matter through energies that are constantly transforming.

We have so far spoken only of what in Einsteinian terms we could define as space, but ... what about time? I believe the balance continues, and allows us to suspect the existences of a "Non time" balancing the classic concept of time. Scientific discoveries tell us that there is more anti-matter than matter, so we can deduce the probable existence of "Non-time".

To conclude, what is important is that we are more convinced of the existence of cosmic frequencies that I see as natural signs or instruments or resources from other dimensions, that are in permanent interaction and about which we know little or nothing but which we can somehow use to our advantage.

The growth of a flower and its life span give us a temporal idea of physical existence, but equally reveal a biological evolution whereby matter "is born again", so that it is plausible to think of the existence of a kind of invisible motor that propels and energizes life into the form in which we know it.

Before leaving these speculations regarding the God, Universe, Biology relationship we should answer questions, some of which are awkward, about whether, in the light of science and technology, it will be possible to know God. The idea is to move forward, to broaden our conscience, to energize it so as to reach those energy levels that might allow us simultaneously to enjoy a greater understanding of the properties of that energy nucleus that we can define as God.

Access to these frequencies enriches us spiritually, mentally and materially in many ways. That is why I have an ethical obligation to transmit, with respect, this knowledge to other people, and to foster, among other things, a broader awareness of healing.

To resume, I am absolutely convinced that there is an overall universal energy authority, existing in various dimensions, infinite in space and existing outside of time (in a non-time). This would explain the perpetuation of evolutionary development at a biological level, as is confirmed by the growing understanding that humans have of their environment thanks to science. On the contrary, and assuming that energy is always information, we can conclude that our knowledge of that energy is at very basic levels, yet is nevertheless headed towards our determination to get ever closer to knowledge of it.

Where would I place human faith and beliefs in this area? Faith is a tool incorporated in humans since we have existed, that is to say for millennia, even preceding the religions. It is something that is in some way genetic, that makes us search for something above us so that we can be secure in the sense that our cycle of life is protected.

In my medical proceedings I always try to establish mental associations between vibration energies and the superior energy levels of each person. As a result, it is also possible to understand in this way those cures that are caused by faith and by prayer, which are common to various religions and cultures, some of which seek to connect via these energy tools to the superior levels our ancestors are endowed with.

Obviously, if we are to ascend to greater heights we will find new and unknown things. My way of conceiving God is therefore logical and is based on the idea that "He is the energy motor that intelligently perpetuates biological evolution". God therefore is converted for me into something more tangible and reasonable than what my Catholic roots allowed me to see when I was a teenager in Austria.

When all is said and done, there is the possibility that we humans can distance ourselves from the religious and spiritual roots of our existence and chase after a fresh new concept, wholly unfettered with traditional contexts, that allows us to gain a greater awareness with which to maximize our potential for our own benefit and the benefit of everything around us. Humanity, somehow, needs to break the ties of religions as a point of cultural disengagement and to seek a new, genuinely universal idea to help us open our minds to the fullest extent in order to make possible the impossible.

MY FIRST ENCOUNTER WITH THESE ENERGIES

Of course, my Hellenistic formation in a country that made Catholicism the seal of its national identity prevented me from even beginning to think of these conclusions during my adolescence in Salzburg. Yet that city was nevertheless the scene of a deeply disturbing and at the same time wonderful experience that would undoubtedly change my life, even though for many years I could provide no reasonable explanation to that mountain of lights that suddenly, like an avalanche, exploded into my room.

I was thirteen years old at the time. I was sleeping in a small room in my father's house when suddenly an intense flash of light made me get out of bed full of fear and disbelief. It was a very strange situation, and my astonishment at that succession of white lights that seemed to grow with every second was then followed by an uncontrollable sensation of heat and of involuntary vibrations throughout my body.

My astonishment was such that, having no way of explaining to myself what had happened, I gave up on the possibility of telling anyone at home about that vision of light and that heat that at times had seemed unbearable. So I chose to do the most logical and reasonable thing a thirteen-year-old could decide to do: I made what

I had experienced into my secret, so that only within myself was I able to return, again and again, to any glimmer of meaning that could help me understand that incomprehensible event.

My secret continued as such even after I realized that that sensation of heat was becoming something constant. I began to experience frequent bouts of heat that would not disappear. They were most evident when those close to me somehow felt that I was transmitting this heat to them. Also, it was most intense in the early morning, between four and six. That is possibly the reason why I have always got up very early ever since, and it is a custom which is accompanied by a constant sensation of thirst caused by the heat.

To begin with, my experience was also followed by a mild depression, but this did not last. Of course, from the time ten years ago that I began to understand the world of frequency vibrations, the depressions have been more moderate, almost imperceptible, and as far as I can tell, they precede the moments when I think I am receiving the electric charges.

Effectively, ten years ago I was getting more frequent depressions, and as the depression began, I sensed a sort of "charge" that entered my body giving me a sort of shiver: my body 'bristled". However, once the experience was over I had no headache and from that fleeting sense of depression I passed to an indescribable happiness that ended in tears. It was like an ecstasy that could last four or five minutes. Today I can still repeat this ecstasy with my mind, though not, of course, with the same intensity as when it happens unexpectedly.

I need, of course, to explain to the reader the mention I have made in these paragraphs to matters relating to a mild depression. This is far from being a pattern of depression of a clinical type related to bipolar disorders, nor anything of the kind. In fact I am not given to suffer from depression, and luckily I consider myself to be a happy person.

What I want to share with my readers is that, at that time, the "charge" would occur without my being aware of it, accompanied by a mild depression which I naturally associated with the depression experienced by millions of people in normal everyday situations of stress brought on by the environment in which we live.

Then soon I understood that that moderate and fleeting depressionhad nothing to do with this, but that it occurred after episodes of loneliness. In fact, the loneliness was the stronger of the two. In conclusion, that energy charge occurred at times when I was alone, which confronted me with an infinite loneliness, not in this case mine but that of human beings faced with situations such as death and passage to another dimension.

I hope that the reader will now understand more easily how that loneliness was followed by a depression that only left me when I experienced that invisible energy charge. It is a phenomenon of loneliness that becomes a depression that I escape from completely thanks to that charge. Indeed, after the charge I feel infinitely accompanied, the world changes for me, I feel that it is completely new and I feel my strengths renewed. It is like a rebirth that allows me to start afresh with more enthusiasm than ever.

This experience that I have described for you has not been very frequent of late, only occurring every two or three months. Despite this, I believe that that sensation of ecstasy, which I would not compare to the altered consciousness of a real trance, is related to the experience I had when I was thirteen, in other words I am wholly convinced that all this is related to that vibration, to that charge of vibration energy that I received in my room as an adolescent in Austria. Of course, the luminosity of that experience has never again been as intense as on that occasion.

The sense of wellbeing and balance brought on by that energy when it arrives even makes me look forward to those moments, and this is also something I connect to the fact that I have no fear of death. I do fear pain, but not the transition involved in shedding the known material world. I am sure this is related to my conviction that there is a "life beyond" charged with intense and pleasant energies about which at present we know very little.

For me it's about a delight. Frankly, if people knew the dimension of this delight not only would they not fear the experience but they would even desire it. Of course my delight with the energy charge I receive cannot be compared to what I felt the first time. Then, and I humbly admit this, I experienced a fear that only left me many years later when it transformed into delight, which is what I would hope many others could learn to experience.

On the other hand, this energy charge is something that only happens when I am on my own and without my necessarily thinking these thoughts. At the level of my body, what I feel with the ecstasy is indescribable and brings tears and a delight I cannot put into words, always with great happiness that is also difficult to describe. Whatever the case, it is an experience that can happen at any moment, even very early in the morning.

In any case, what strikes me at those moments is a sense of happiness greater, for example, that that I experience when one of my patients overcomes cancer. In these cases my eyes also moisten, but when I experience an ecstasy such as I have described, this crying is stronger, uncontrollable and inevitable, however much I might want to contain it. It is undoubtedly something very strange.

It is also worthwhile to explain to the reader that I don't relate the reduced frequency of these experiences to my work capacity, i.e. my ability to carry out my therapies. The energy charge, the "raw material" of my work, does not specifically depend on those wonderful experiences which have given me a sense of my mission in this world, the aim of my life and my *raison d'être*.

CONCLUSION

In reference to the above, I tend to believe that we should all work towards identifying and accepting the possibilities offered us by the universe and to direct our lives along paths of permanent learning until and insofar as we are enabled to by that spirituality that is somehow part of us all.

We can assume, in this first phase of analysis, that this spiritual element is somehow a kind of tutor that we each have within us, and which guides us on a mission about which we know nothing, and that the best thing is always to incorporate into our conception of life a series of values that allow us to live in harmony with ourselves, in other words, within the rules and styles of conduct that help us find physical, mental and spiritual wellbeing and to avoid states where one or other field of life prevails over another.

When I look at ordinary people and compare them with personalities who have shaped history, it occurs to me that many of these personalitieswere guided, for good or for evil, in a different way from ordinary people. This is in no way something we should regret, particularly if we compare ourselves with those who have been guided correctly to bring to the world knowledge that humanity had previously lacked.

What I wish to underline here is that perhaps we can all obtain and use the information from those other dimensions so that they help us achieve holistic growth, that is, growth that is integral insofar as it allows us to achieve spiritual, mental and physical balance to underpin the success of the life plan that we set out for ourselves.

If we achieve this fullness of life over a long period, hopefully for most of our life, it will mean that all we do for ourselves and for others will also be re-vindicated, as this is the fruit of the great potential we have in our hands once we opt to believe in reincarnation and in all its possible aspects, projections and manifestations.

I must admit it is not easy for anyone to accept reincarnation when for the first time we are faced with the possibility that it is this phenomenon that guides our lives. This is all the more true in the modern context of globalization, which tends to homogenize the conception of an exclusively material world that attempts to ignore spirituality and limit it to the individual conscience of each person. It is also true because of the effects of religious activism, born also of intercultural suspicions, which motivates each civilization to defend its faith.

When, as is increasingly visible in our time, we are faced with different religions, beliefs, religious practices and dogmas of interpretation of each religious sentiment, we can understand that a profusion of information of all kinds is circulated on a subject such as reincarnation which undoubtedly causes an explosion of religious and philosophical fanaticisms which only contribute to increase confusion when we attempt to approach the subject.

To conclude, it is not easy to struggle with an idea of this kind when many countries of the world are involved in political and religious conflicts that relate to the interpretation of their past, that is to say, committed to preconceived interpretations of their history.

The exercise of re-thinking history is sometimes useful, when it is a question of scrutinizing the legacy of men like Jean-Jacques Rousseau and Immanuel Kant, eighteenth century philosophers who proposed the basis of a new political thinking upon which Europe erected its democratic systems nearly two-hundred and fifty years later. Nearly three centuries had to pass before the Western world could understand the extent of that revolution in human thought. Rousseau, particularly, allows us to deduce how he transformed the minds of many people when he molded his philosophical thought in a world that held as absolute truth—and as such perennial and immutable—the political order derived from the monarchic absolutism of Old Europe, at the time dominated by the *ancien régime*.

Few today will deny that the history of the pre-democratic revolution in the political sphere was written in the eighteenth century, yet despite globalization and technology, the case of Rousseau shows us that the argument is not yet won for those who want to believe in modern democracy in the twenty-first century.

By analogy we can state that the scientific and medical moment of today is still at a pre-revolutionary stage, in a state needing profound change if we want to see new steps in the evolution of man.

What is important is to highlight that what we want is for people to learn to interpret the relativity of things, which includes reinterpretation of medical science, and for this it is fundamental to abandon rigid, inflexible schemes as regards the concepts of sickness and health, so that perhaps we may be able to accept more fully, with more awareness, the substitute, complementary or alternative role that other therapies should have in curing the various pathologies, some of which therapies are becoming more prevalent due to some consequences of our century's life-styles.

What is needed for that revolution in the world of medicine to be viable? The most important pre-requisite for this change to be achieved undoubtedly rests, as with any revolution, on a change of mentality. For this to happen, patients need a greater and better knowledge of their rights, as a means of gaining clearer criteria about the evolution of their health, their chances of improvement according to the therapy they choose, the collateral effects of therapies, the long-term consequences, the length of convalescence, their symptomatology, their treatment and recuperation, whether or not they will become drug-dependent, the costs of the procedures and the degree of participation they will themselves need to have in the cure of theirdisease.

TESTIMONIES OF SOME PATIENTS

To illustrate my experience of treating various diseases with very different patients, I feel it is logical that I leave some space to a few testimonies from those who were able, thanks to my therapy, to overcome difficult diagnoses. All these patients had for years been treated with conventional medicine, but without success. It is certainly not my intention to question the traditional treatments given to these patients, but to highlight the importance of opening our minds to new healing perspectives. Three patients managed this very effectively, and they have generously agreed to tell their stories.

RUTH MURILLO, DIAGNOSED WITH GLOMUS YUGULAR

"The first time I visited Dr. Willy Frinta was towards the end of November of 2006. My decision to attend his consulting room was in a way my last hope of a cure for my glomusyugular, a rare disease and one so difficult to diagnose that it is almost always detected late. The symptoms are truly unbearable: intense headaches, blurred vision, loss of hearing in the right ear, dysphonia, loss of balance, facial numbness and nausea. What most worried me, however, in addition to the loss of hearing, was the increasing difficulty I had to speak, because the pain was very intense every time I made the effort for my words to be heard. In fact I felt that I was losing my voice. It was very hoarse, as when someone has a very bad 'flu, so with this and the great pain, I was forced to avoid speaking whenever possible, and this all was very depressing. The idea of losing my voice was very stressful, all the more so because I am an English teacher, and if I lose my voice I lose my livelihood for life, and this, quite frankly, terrified me.

My clinical picture during those two long years, from 2005 to 2006, was not connected to any other pathology by any of the specialists who treated me, despite the fact that the case history indicated a relationship to a strong knock I had had in 2005 when part of a desk fell on my face.

I was given audiometry tests when I noticed that the knock had made me a bit deaf, and these confirmed that the deafness was getting worse and I was also suffering increasing facial pain and headaches that even affected my mobility. In fact, a sudden movement or the simple act of bending to pick something up caused me great pain.

The ear and throat specialists who treated me during those years were unable to stop the pain or to give a precise diagnosis of the disease. In my effort and those of the doctors to overcome my afflictions I had a nose operation which caused me great post-operative pain and a device was embedded in my ear; neither treatment was of any use whatsoever.

Finally, in October 2006, a facial magnetic resonance test gave the final diagnosis of glomusyugular, an ailment characterized by the growth of a tumor situated between the jugular and carotid arteries, which puts pressure on them and produces intense pain, deafness and dysfunction in the system of ducts of the ear, nose and throat.

In addition to the diagnosis I was given an option to halt the tumor and restore some of my function, my speech among others, which was unthinkable for me. According to the medical team, I would have to have an operation that would last an average of 12 hours and which could still leave me with facial paralysis for life. Of course, the results of the magnetic resonance test and the possibility of losing mobility in my face caused me deep despair and depression, which ended up affecting my sleep. Insomnia, caused not only by the pain but also by the anguish that all this was giving me, began to cause havoc in my life. To combat the pain I had to take ever greater doses of painkillers which gave me a sensation of impotence in relation to the disease.

In these conditions I heard about Dr. Willy Frinta's *healing* therapy. I was told about it by a friend living in Miami who a few days previously had seen, on a Spanish language TV programme in Florida, how Dr. Frinta uses non-conventional energies to control therapeutically a wide range of diseases. I arrived without much hope, motivated only by the vague idea that perhaps I should not refuse to try something different in the fight against my illness and determined not to allow myself to be operated, particularly as the anticipated outcome was that it would not heal the facial paralysis that was getting worse every day.

I cannot forget the day I began my treatment. It was the 21st of November, 2006. Before the first therapy session, and with my test results in front of him, Dr. Frinta was cautious about his chances of improving my condition. His openness about how long the treatment could last was something that helped me not to be disillusioned that the cure would not be as quick as in my state of anxiety I ferventlyhoped.

In fact, his forecast that I would probably not notice an improvement until after the fifth or sixth session proved to be literally the case. Thus it was that I began to notice a general improvement after little more that a month and a half, so that I began the year 2007 with renewed hope of a complete cure.

What most astonished me about the therapy was the intermittent sensation of hot and cold that took hold of me. I felt in fact as though a metal plate was inside my head, and also had the impression that the aroma of the consulting room remained with me for several days. But unlike what normally happened with other patients, I found it difficult to sleep during therapy, and if I managed it it only lasted fractions of a second. Of course, something that also helped me to persevere with the treatment when I had just begun it was the testimonies that I heard in the consulting room from other patients, as also the improvement that I noticed in many of them from one week to the next.

As I got better, the sessions became more spaced out, from weekly to fortnightly and then every 20 days, and I went to them with my mother. I am very grateful to her for the support she gave me in those very difficult months, but when they were over I noticed that I had not only improved generally but that my morale had improved as well. The pressure in the face, the headaches and the nausea slowly disappeared, and my voice regained its usual tone. I sounded as I had always sounded and I no longer had that pain in my vocal chords every time I tried to pronounce a word.

Today, three years after that experience, I have nothing but words of thanks, first to God, of course, and then to Dr. Frinta, to whom I owe my recuperation, which was not only physical but also, I would say without exaggeration, mental and spiritual. I can in fact say that since then my life has changed. I have an unshakable faith in the possibilities life offers us. I live differently to how I used to live, for now my hope and my faith that there are energies that transcend us are things that fill me with infinite peace and have made me appreciate life more than ever.

When I agreed to tell my story in this book that Dr. Frinta has decided to publish I realized immediately that my witness could help other people who, like myself, had lost hope that a cure was possible with healing therapies. Today I can proudly say that life has turned full circle. I have improved from every point of view, I now value much more all that I have around me and so far as is possible I try to help people. And all of this has been a blessing in my life, and the least I can do is to share it with each one of you."

MÉLIDA GALINDO DE SALAZAR, DIAGNOSED WITH GANGRENE

"Although I had known for a long time about the astonishing results obtained by Dr. Willy Frinta's treatments, it was not until 2006 that I discovered the enormous possibilities we have, as his patients, to recover from an impressive range of diseases, many of them with terrible diagnoses, thanks to the mysterious energies of his wonderful hands.

I met Dr. Frinta in the mid 1990s in Chia. My memories of him are of an infinitely affable and simple man whom I almost always saw surrounded by dozens of sick people, most of them children, almost all of them poor, over whom he approached his hands as he slowly went round the circle of those men, women and children in the courtyard of the school of Stella Matutina.

Of course, years had passed and I had lost contact with him, and I only looked for him again when I was sent as an emergency to hospital in the Clínica Cardio-Infantil, in Bogotá, with an unbearable pain in my right leg, accompanied by a reddening and rapid accumulation of pus in the ten sores that had formed, particularly on the ankle. I soon learned, and the doctors confirmed this, that because of my history of diabetes discovered in a routine examination in 1990, I had to have my leg amputated in just a few days' time as the only solution for a gangrenous ulcer which, if not controlled with the operation, could soon lead to acute septicemia that would probably kill me.

For the twenty-two days I was in hospital, the idea of losing my leg was something I could not at all assimilate. I so wanted to be cured that I could not believe there was no alternative to that of losing my mobility and being confined to a wheel chair, perhaps for the rest of my life, with all that that implied for someone as active as I still am today.

I knew little about diabetes, for the disease had been diagnosed as an a-symptomatic picture. I did not suffer from thirst, nor from urinary problems that might have made me suspect the presence of that disease in my organism. In fact a glycemia test in 1990 was what revealed high blood sugar levels, 450 to be precise, so that I began the necessary diet.

Despite these precautions, the swelling in my foot, the redness, the pain I suffered more and more intensely and the appearance of bruising around the ankle and on the foot itself, affected by a cut that would not heal, all meant that I had to be sent to hospital. For the doctors who looked after me at the Clínica Cardio-Infantil, the only possible solution in order to avoid the spread of the gangrene was the amputation of my foot, but because time went by while I refused the operation, the condition got worse and the diagnosis became more terrible still: not just the foot but the leg as far as the knee would have to be amputated.

At this point I remembered about Dr. Frinta. I asked the surgeons for two weeks' delay and immediately began to search for Dr. Frinta via the many people he had treated and cured. I was lucky enough to find him, I asked him for an appointment and we agreed that treatment would begin immediately. When I left the hospital with the aim of starting treatment with Dr. Frinta I had ten suppurating sores, they all had pus and I could see that my foot was practically rotting. While I had been in hospital they had given me high doses of antibiotics and painkillers which made no improvement. I had nausea, giddiness and fainting fits which showed, according to the doctors, that the infection was continuing its unstoppable course.

After I turned to Dr. Frinta, things changed faster than I had thought. The first time I went to his consulting room the foot was so big I could not put on a shoe; I had to put it in a plastic bag to stop it getting even more infected. When he saw me he stopped the antibiotic, removed the bandages and, in a decision that I judged bold, he stopped the painkillers as well, which I accepted with good grace because of the improvement that I could see in the patients who came with me to the therapies.

I remember fondly how my daughter María Mercedes came to see me in my room on the day after my first session. She was fairly skeptical as to whether I had chosen the right path, but when she saw me she could not believe the improvement shown by my foot. With the first therapies the sores started to heal and to begin with they suppurated yellow matter but then that became water, from which I understood that the infection was disappearing as the pus came out of the sores on its own. Of course my confidence rose to such an extent that, in agreement with Dr. Frinta, we decided to continue the treatment for some six months, after which the foot was completely healthy, my mobility was total, the sores had scarred over completely and the leg and foot were back to their normal size.

I will also never forget what I felt during those sessions. In the consulting room a strange sensation of relaxation, tranquility and pleasant drowsiness gave me an experience that was different to everything else. The gentle heat I received when his hands approached to a maximum of 20 cm of the affected areas calmed me more than one could imagine. My thirst after the therapies could last several hours, but I always felt a certain itchiness that showed that the foot was healing.

Almost two years have now passed since I chose vibration *healing*, and I can assure you that I am a completely healthy person, for which I am profoundly thankful, to God first, and of course to Dr. Frinta, to whom I owe the fact that today I can have a normal life next to my daughters and grand-children."

ALBERTO MARTÍNEZ, DIAGNOSED WITH CANCER OF THE BLADDER

"The images I saw on the computer screen could not have been worse, on that October day in 2008 when I was first given a cystoscopy, an intra-urethral examination where the doctor introduces, through the urethral duct of the penis, a tiny probe that reaches the bladder in order to search for signs of tumors and other tissue anomalies. Indeed, a series of red points contrasting with the pink tissue of the urethra confirmed the presence in my organism of cancer of the bladder. I had decided to have that test on the recommendation of a doctor friend to whom I had turned for help after having discovered with horror... that I have, on this occasion, considerable bleeding and no urine.

The images on the computer indicated the presence of six tumors, so I was immediately operated to remove the cancerous nodules. However, the result of the surgery was worse than expected: a total of fourteen malignant tumors were removed from the urethral duct. I was prescribed a treatment with specific drugs that, in addition to cleaning the tissues completely, were intended to prevent the recurrence of the cancer. But the disease returned sooner than expected and with the next cystoscopy, two months after the operation, they found four tumors, which confused the doctors who had hoped that by then there would be none at all. I was given another operation, with results that were again disheartening. Instead of the four cancerous nodules the doctors found six malignant malformations sticking obstinately to the walls of the urethra and the bladder.

It was obvious that I was suffering from a very aggressive form of cancer, which was confirmed as soon as I was ready for a third examination of diagnostic images: six more tumors had quickly appeared, so there was no choice but to perform a third operation, and the doctors no longer held out hope of a recovery. My life expectancy depended on how well I was able to survive however many operations would be needed to remove the cancerous tumors.

It was then that I decided to rebel against the conventional treatment that for patients such as myself would end up being fruitless and an eventual metastasis that would clearly be terminal. I began to pin my hopes on all sorts of alternative treatments, includingapitherapy, whichinduces bee stings in the affected areas. I abandoned this after two months given that the cancer was progressing, with seven tumors in addition to the six detected in the previous cystoscopy further complicating a panorama that seemed to have no escape.

This being the case, I heard towards the end of 2008 about vibration *healing*. I went to Dr. Frinta's consulting room, and having looked carefully over my clinical history he said something I will remember as long as I live: 'Alberto, give me twelve sessions. You'll have to be very disciplined, and then you'll need to have another cystoscopy'. His confidence that he would cure me proved prophetic. After the first four sessions, and having stopped the drugs I had been on, I was surprised to see that the urethral dysfunction commonly known as urinary urgency—a condition leading to incontinence— had disappeared, and that many of the symptoms of the disease had been considerably reduced. My trust in the treatment became total, even though after the first two sessions I was exhausted and so weak I could not get out of bed, yet this seemed a natural response to the therapy.

After fourteen sessions, Dr. Frinta decided the treatment could not continue without a new cystoscopy. The test was needed so that decisions could be made about what had happened to the tumors and how they had responded to the therapy. 'Don't come back without the exam results,' said Dr. Frinta in a friendly but firm manner. So I decided to have the test done in Bogotá's Central Military Hospital. I still have fresh in my memory the image of the doctor when he read the history before doing the test. Considering that this test is an essential tool for following the evolution of the cancer, and that eight months had passed since the previous test, his complaint sounded like a scolding. He warned me that I and I alone was responsible if the disease had reached an irreversible stage, he then carried out the test. I remember that it took a bit longer than usual, partly because he was determined to find indications of the presence of tumors in the urethral duct. After almost forty minutes the computer screen showed nothing but healthy, pink walls, without scarring or anything to suggest the recurrence of the disease.

That was one of the happiest days of my life. The doctor, half disbelieving and half embarrassed, accepted that I was better. And with the test results under my arm I went back to Dr. Frinta in May of 2009. From my expression Dr. Frinta guessed that things were going well. "You look pretty pleased," he said when he saw me come in. 'You're cured, aren't you?' 'Yes, it seems I am,' I agreed with a joy I will never forget."

INDEX OF DISEASES

GLOSSARY OF THERAPIES

Given the great number of therapies and techniques that are considered in the realm of alternative medicine, patients and their families are usually faced with a saturation of information that complicates understanding about which type of medicine is valid for those who choose not to follow conventional methods. And although the main theme of this work is vibration energy *healing*, it is logical that we should help to bring clarity regarding the most common procedures of what is globally known as alternative medicine.

ANTHROPOSOPHIC MEDICINE

As its name says, this medicine is based on a holistic concept of the human being, so it supports the thesis that therapies should not focus on the body alone, which would distance them from the human sphere. For specialists in anthroposophic medicine, all disease is the result of an imbalance of the so-called polar functions of the organism, i.e. the anabolic functions (such as metabolism, nutrition and reproduction) and the catabolizing functions (comprising the nervous system and the five senses). Good health is the result of keeping these in balance, and as a result it requires substances whose main aim is to restore this harmony. The therapist looks for the cause of the sickness and thereby explores its cure.

AROMATHERAPY

This is a technique based on the extraction of essential oils derived from aromatic plants and spices with limited physical, mental and emotional curative effects. It uses more that eighty essences and is an area of herbology, but unlike this, the essences are not ingested but are inhaled or applied to the skin.

AYURVEDIC MASSAGE

This technique, related to Indian medicine based on a global vision of man, aims to heal both body and spirit. The massage does not cure, but it strengthens the body and restores the positive energy it needs for good physical form and mental wellbeing.

CHROMOTHERAPY

A therapy based on the supposedly curative use of the energy of light emitted by different colours with the aim of unleashing in the organism psychological and chemical reactions capable of helping both diagnosis of disease and their treatment. Its curative effects have been questioned, though it cannot be denied that some people show improvement resulting from the deep profiles of suggestion which bring some patients to sample this type of techniques.

FLORAL REMEDIES: BACH, CALIFORNIA AND OTHERS

A technique that uses thirty-eight floral essences to treat diseases that are caused, according to its advocates, by profound maladjustments in the emotional and mental balance of human beings, so that these essences are able to produce moods that induce curing and improvements in certain types of illness, particularly those whose evolution towards more advanced states can be associated with stress-related disorders, anxiety or with depressive profiles that allow the appearance of certain pathologies to be somatized.

HYDROTHERAPY

This is based on the therapeutic use of water in any state, form or temperature. This therapy, one of the oldest in the history of medicine, has a wide range of palliative and curative properties for treating a wide range of sicknesses based on water's ability to induce changes in the human organism according to its pressure or the variations of heat with which it can be applied in different conditions. It is an accepted fact that hydrotherapy can be very useful to eliminate toxins and inflammation and to reduce muscular tensions. It can be applied with frictions, compresses, inhalations, immersion baths, specific washes and any other type of contact. These can help with relaxation, reduce pain and activate circulation.

HOMEOPATHY

This conceives medical treatment on the basis of minute doses of substances that, were they given to healthy individuals in greater quantities, would provoke symptoms similar to those they aim to combat. Samuel Hahnemann, considered to have been the father of homeopathy, based his approach on the principle that "like cures like", and that "the effect of a medication is inversely proportional to its quantity". The main characteristic of homeopathic preparations is their innocuousness as regards collateral effects. This is because its compounds are so diluted that their presence is almost infinitesimal in the medication, so the healing processes tend to be longer, though the lack of secondary effects compensates for this.

IRIDOLOGY

More than a therapy, we can say that iridology is a technique for diagnosing diseases based on the observation of the iris through a magnifying glass, on the basis that this part of the eye is different for each individual, which makes it a kind of imprint that reveals a person's general state of health. This procedure is still practised by country doctors in China with some success, so it is well supported by the country's authorities as a means to lower the costs of diagnosis.

KINESIOLOGY

Medical and therapeutic procedure based on the study of human movement from a physical point of view. Kinesiology can be a useful diagnostic method, particularly from the tracing and analysis of a patient's muscular movement.

METAMORPHIC MASSAGE

Focused on those parts of the human organism that are first formed in the uterus during the embryonic stage, metamorphic massage is based on self-healing and on the idea that the body is endowed with a vital impulse that gives strength and health to the organism. This technique seeks to activate prenatal energy with the aim of unleashing chain reactions by stimulating cell memory, so it concentrates on massaging the feet, arms and head.

MUSIC THERAPY

Used basically as a complementary therapy in treating certain conditions related to mental and behavioral alterations, this technique is based on music as a tool for controlling feelings and emotions. Music therapy is also very functional in treating motor and cognitive disabilities in children.

NATUROPATHY

Although this is a naturist treatment of disease, it follows a physical-chemical perspective so is no doubt one of the treatments that are closest to conventional medicine. Many of the drugs produced by the world's big laboratories are in fact no more than syntheses of the active principles present in many plants used in naturopathy. This medicine aims to attack physical and psychological disorders affecting human beings. It uses complementary diets, exercises, massages and thermal baths, and opposes the consumption of sugars, fats and alcohol.

OSTEOPATHY

This is a paramedical practice based on the thesis that the great majority of diseases are caused by systemic structural disorders that have repercussions in other organs by means of chain reactions that can only be corrected with manipulation of joints, muscles and entrails, which are able to restore arterial, venous and lymphatic circulation. Treatment seeks to revitalize blood circulation and in this way restore a normal degree of mobility to a damaged joint.

PHYTOTHERAPY

This is undoubtedly one of the most common therapies in the world of alternative medicine, and is based on the idea that health can be re-established with the use of vegetable remedies, extracts of roots, leaves, cuttings, flowers, seeds and fruits. Phytotherapy is in some senses a branch of herbal medicine that believes that nature contains a species able to cure every human illness. Normally it is believed that so-called curative plants can be useful in treating some digestive, pancreatic, pulmonary, circulatory and nervous diseases, among others.

REFLEXOLOGY

This is a technique that applies massage to feet and hands as a means to unleash in the organism impulses that have curative properties. This type of medicine is based on the fact that the nerves in feet and hands are like terminals that are connected to the organs that affect their functions. Reflexology holds that stimulating specific points in the feet and hands of patients can bring about healing.

REIKI

This is a medical technique that originated in Japan that seeks to balance the body energy of human beings on the physical, mental, emotional and spiritual levels. Therapists transmit their energy to patients without in fact touching them during the therapy, and they thus relieve and restore the levels of energy in such a way that healing reactions are activated. This technique is often used in treatment of rheumatism and arthritis and induces the states of deep relaxation that are needed for the therapy. It causes significant exhaustion in professionals who practice it as they really do transmit their energies to the patients.

SHIATSU

This is a technique developed in China which incorporates Western traditions such as osteopathy and chiropractic. The therapist exerts pressure with fingers, as also with elbows and knees, and is thus able to detect the blockage points that cause illness. Shiatsu holds that energies follow the meridians, so it is able to relieve headache and back pain and other illnesses such as digestive and nervous problems.

SOPHROLOGY

This is a combination of relaxation techniques aimed at achieving controlled alteration of states of consciousness with the aim of reestablishing the mental and corporal balance of human beings. It was created in the 1960s by the Colombian neuro-psychiatrist Alfonso Caycedo Lozano. It differs from hypnosis in that sophrology keeps the person awake. For several decades, in addition to its therapeutic use in medicine, sophrology has been used in clinical psychology with very promising results for the treatment of many emotional and behavioral dysfunctions that can trigger certain diseases.

TAI CHI AND QI GONG

Qi Gong brings together the therapeutic effects of energy gymnastics and relaxation, based on the use of the so-called vital force or Qi, which is a technique taken from Chinese medicine. Curing energies are unleashed with this procedure, unblocking tension points that, according to this therapy, are the cause of many complaints. As for Tai Chi, it combines the strength and grace of many movements associated with the ancient techniques of combat, which are also complemented with concentration and breathing practices that can reduce depression and anxiety.

THALASSOTHERAPY

This is a therapy that uses the curative properties of the sea, and the technique derives its name from "talasa", the Greek word for sea, and "terapia", healing. Scientifically, thalassotherapy was developed in Great Britain in the middle of the nineteenth century, with studies that corroborated the efficacy of the treatments, which had been used since antiquity in an empirical way. With proper medical supervision, thalassotherapy can prevent and heal certain pathologies. It acts on the bases of three aspects: salt water, sea air and climate, with their specific components of marine temperature and humidity.

YOGA

Though not properly a therapy but an integral relaxation technique, yoga's curative properties are well known. Relaxed states give people sensations of peacefulness and mental concentration that are complemented by the greater and better physical flexibility obtained from the practice of some six hundred positions that help to activate muscles that otherwise are very seldom used, and this causes natural massages that relax other muscles, tendons, bones and joints.

EYE YOGA

This therapy is used to improve eyesight on the basis of stimulating a series of fluted muscles that surround the eye. The exercises performed by these muscles, along with light stimulation, help to optimize the blood irrigation of the eye, improving oxygenation and the patient's optical responses.

COMPENDIUM OF SCIENTIFIC TERMS

Allopathic: The word refers in general terms to all that is dealt with in medicine by conventional means (Faculty medicine).

Radiesthesia: The discovery, by means of a pendulum, of "extra-sensory" responses.

Holistic: This is a global concept of a situation, in this case of medicines (Aristotle and metaphysics).

Radio isotopes: Refers to the radioactivity of an isotope.

Supernatural: Events that lack any explanation.

Extra-sensory: Direct or indirect handling where the human mind gives unconscious energy commands to a receptor.

Action potentials: Electric impulse that travels through the membrane of a nerve.

Metabolism: Biochemical reactions of a general nature that occur in cells.

Incorrupt: State of non-deterioration of a body, keeping intact its internal properties.

Immunological system: System that contemplates and manages the organism's defenses in every way.

Streptococcus: Gram-positive spherical bacterium

Staphylococcus: Gram-positive bacterium

Thermographic camera: Technology for observing the thermic alterations of a living body by means of an infra-red lens.

Ischemia: Transitory lack of blood (oxygen) in blood vessels.

Clot: When blood elements like blood platelets, etc., become compacted and form a thrombus.

Endometrium: Tissue that covers the uterine cavity.

BIBLIOGRAPHY

Bendit, J., and P. Bendit, *The Etheric Body of Man: The Bridge of Consciousness,* Theosophical Publishing House, Weathon, Illinois, 1977.

Cerminara, G., *Many Mansions: The Edgar Cayce Story and Reincarnation,* New American Library, Inc., New York, 1950.

Dossey, L., *Beyond Illness: Discovery The Experience Health,* New Science Library-Shambala Publications Inc., Boston and London, 1984.

Gerber, R., *La CuraciónEnergética. La revolucionariamedicinavibracional. Nuevasalternativasparasanar.* IntermedioedicionesRobinBook, 1993.

Greenhouse, H., *The Astral Journey,* Avon Books, New York, 1974.

Hay, L., *You Can Heal Your Life,* Coleman Publishing, Farmingdale, New York, 1984.

Krieger, D., *The Therapeutic Touch: How to Use your Hands to Help or to Heal.* 1979.

Meek, G., *After We Die, ¿What then? Answers to Questions About Life After Death.* Franklin, North Carolina, 1980.

Mesher, A., *A Journey of Love: A Formula for Mastery and Miracles,* Quartus Foundation, Austin, Texas, 1982.

Moore, M., and L. Moore. *The Complete Handbook of Holistic Health,* Prentice-Hall, Inc. Englewood Cliffs, New Jersey, 1983.

Otto, H, and J. Knight, *Dimensions in Holistic Healing: New Frontiers in the Treatment of the Whole Person,* Nelson-Hall, Chicago, 1979.

Oyle, I., *Time, Space, and the Mind, Celestial Arts,* Millbrae, California, 1976.

Perkins, J., *Experience Reincarnation,* Theosophical Publishing House, Weathon, Illinois, 1977.

Rogo, D., *Mind Beyond and Body.* Penguin Books, 1978.

Talbot, M., *Mysticism and the New Physics,* Bantam Books, New York, 1980.

Tansley, D., and Cols., *Dimensions of Radionics: New Technique of Instrumental Distant Healing,* C. W. Daniel Co. Ltd., Essex. 1977.

Tiller, W.,

--- *A Lattice Model of Space and Its Relationship to Multidimensional Physics. The Positive and Negative Space/Time as Conjugate Systems,* in *Future Science,* compiled by White andKrippner, Doubleday & Co. Ltd., Essex, 1977.

--- *Consciousness, Radiation and the Developing Sensory System,* in *The Dimensions of Healing: A Symposium.* Los Gatos, California, 1973.

--- *Radionics: Interface with the Ether-fields,* Health Science Press, Bradford, 1975.

--- *Radionics: Science or Magic – An Holistic Paradigm of Radionics Theory and Practice,* C., Daniel Co. Ltd. Essex, 1982.

--- *Radionics, Radesthesia and Physics,* in *The Varieties of Healing Experience: Exploring Physics Phenomena in Healing.* Los Angeles, California, 1971.

--- *Some Energy Field Observations and Man and Nature,* in *The Kirlian Aura,* compiled by Krippner and Rubin. Garden City, New York, 1974.

Toben, B., *Space-Time and Beyond,* E. P. Dutton & Co., New York, 1975.

Young, M., Agartha: *A Journey to the Stars,* Stillpoint Publishing, Walpole, New Hampshire, 1984.

Wallace, A. and B. Henkin, *The Psychic Healing Book,* Dell Publishing, New York, 1978.

Weymouth, L., *The Electrical Connection* (Part. 1), in New York Magazine, 24th of Novembre of 1980. Pp. 26-47, 44-58.

White, S., *The Unobstructed Universe.* E. P. Dutton & Co., New York, 1940.

INDEX OF THERAPIES

ANTHROPOSOPHIC MEDICINE
AROMATHERAPY
AURICULOTHERAPY
AYURVEDIC MASSAGE
BACH FLOWERS REMEDIES
CHROMOTHERAPY
HYDROTHERAPY
HOMEOPATHY
IRIDOLOGY
KINESIOLOGY
METAMORPHIC TECHNIQUE/MASSAGE
MUSIC THERAPY
NATUROPATHY
OSTEOPATHY
PHYTOTHERAPY
REFLEXOLOGY
REIKI
SHIATSU
SOPHROLOGY
TAI CHI AND QI GONG
THALASSOTHERAPY
YOGA

INDEX OF THERAPIES

ABOUT THE AUTHOR

My name is Wilhelm Frinta, born in Austria. I am a physician and i am living in Colombia since 35 years. I am treating ill people with energy (vibrational medicine) which i have develloped step by step. I wrote a book "Sanación Energética" several years ago in spanish language. therefore i want this book also in english language published

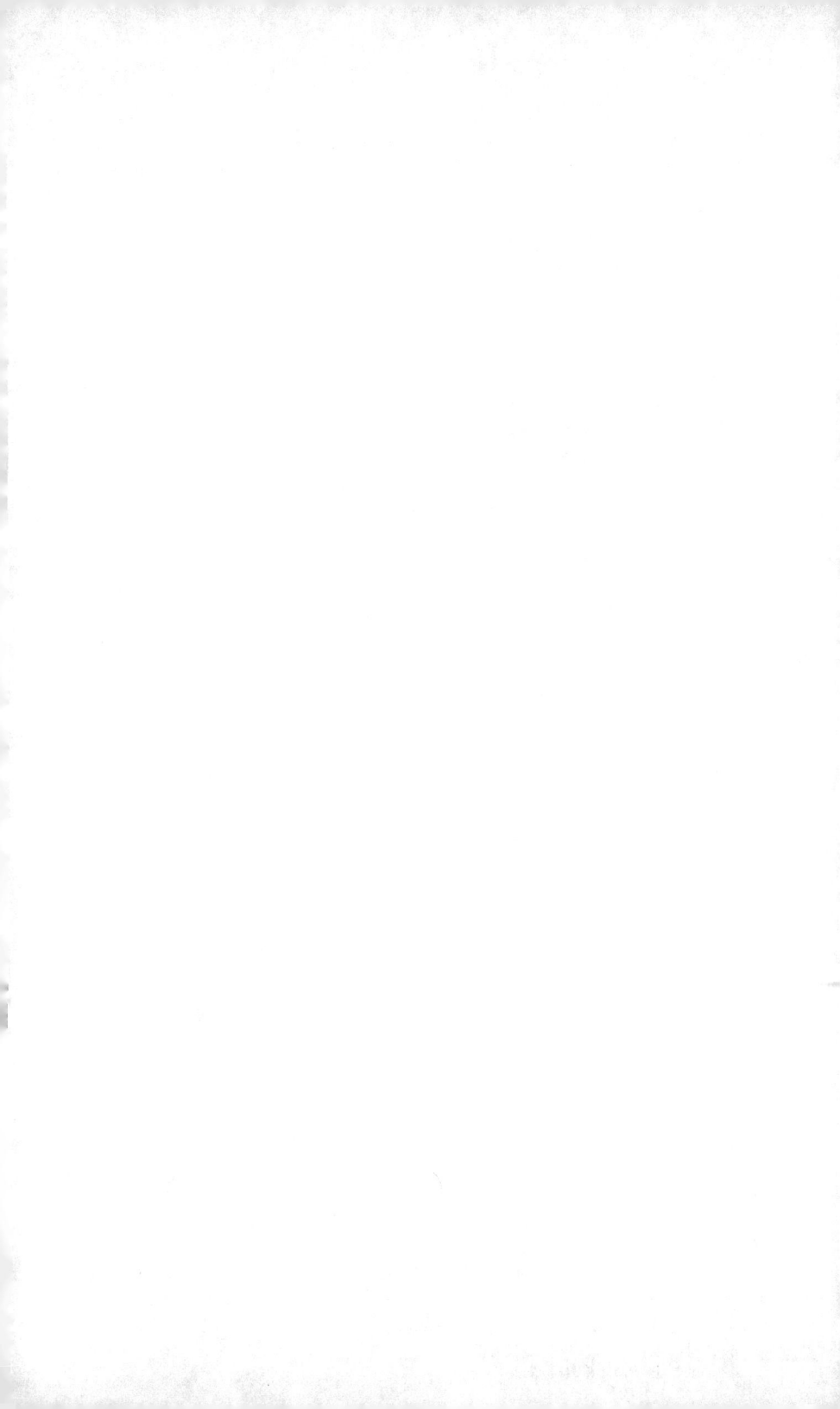

www.ingramcontent.com/pod-product-compliance
Lightning Source LLC
Chambersburg PA
CBHW030945180526
45163CB00002B/704